Drugs of Choice
Drugs of Choice

2019

Selected 2018 Articles from
The Medical Letter on Drugs and Therapeutics®

Published by

The Medical Letter, Inc.
145 Huguenot St.
New Rochelle, New York 10801-7537

800-211-2769
914-235-0500
Fax 914-632-1733
www.medicalletter.org

D0324550

20th Edition

Copyright 2019
(ISSN 1065-6596)
(ISBN 978-0-9846522-0-4)

The Medical Letter Inc.
145 Huguenot St., Ste. 312
New Rochelle, New York 10801-7537

Contents

Tables

Weight Management

Introduction

The Medical Letter, Inc. is a nonprofit organization that publishes critical appraisals of new prescription drugs and comparative reviews of drugs for common diseases in its newsletter, *The Medical Letter on Drugs and Therapeutics*. It is committed to providing objective, practical, and timely information on drugs and treatments of common diseases to help readers make the best decisions for their patients—without the influence of the pharmaceutical industry. The Medical Letter is supported by its readers, and does not receive any commercial support or accept advertising in any of its publications.

Many of our readers know that pharmaceutical companies and their representatives often exaggerate the therapeutic effects and understate the adverse effects of their products, but busy practitioners have neither the time nor the resources to check the accuracy of the manufacturers' claims. Our publication is intended specifically to meet the needs of busy healthcare professionals who want unbiased, reliable, and timely drug information. Our editorial process is designed to ensure that the information we provide represents an unbiased consensus of medical experts.

The editorial process used for *The Medical Letter on Drugs and Therapeutics* relies on a consensus of experts to develop prescribing recommendations. The first draft of an article is prepared by one of our in-house or contributing editors or by an outside expert. This initial draft is edited and sent to our Contributing Editors, to 10-20 other reviewers who have clinical and/or experimental experience with the drug or type of drug or disease under review, to the FDA, and to the first and last authors of all the articles cited in the text. Many critical observations, suggestions, and questions are received from the reviewers and are incorporated into the article during the revision process. Further communication as needed is followed by fact checking and editing to make sure the final appraisal is not only accurate, but also easy to read.

NOTE: The drug costs listed in the tables are based on the pricing information that was available in the month the article was originally published. When the cost of a drug has been updated or added since publication, it is designated as such.

The Medical Letter, Inc. is based in New Rochelle, NY. For more information, go to www.medicalletter.org or call 800-211-2769.

Adult Immunization

Original publication date – May 2018

The US Advisory Committee on Immunization Practices (ACIP) recommends routine use of the following vaccines in adults residing in the US: influenza, tetanus/diphtheria alone (Td) and in combination with acellular pertussis (Tdap), measles/mumps/rubella (MMR), varicella (VAR), herpes zoster (RZV; ZVL), human papillomavirus (HPV), and pneumococcal conjugate (PCV13) and polysaccharide (PPSV23) vaccines. For adults with certain medical conditions or occupational, behavioral, or other risk factors, hepatitis A (HepA), hepatitis B (HepB), meningococcal (MenACWY; MenB), and *Haemophilus influenzae* type b (Hib) vaccines are also recommended.[1] Recommendations for vaccination against seasonal influenza and vaccination of travelers are reviewed separately.[2,3]

VACCINE PREPARATIONS

Inactivated vaccines are prepared from whole or fractional antigenic components of viruses or bacteria. Fractional vaccines are usually either protein- or polysaccharide-based. Protein-based vaccines typically include subunits of microbiologic protein or inactivated bacterial toxins (toxoids). Polysaccharide-based vaccines are generally less immunogenic than protein-based vaccines; they may be conjugated to a protein to increase immune response and enhance immune memory.

Live-attenuated vaccines use a weakened form of the pathogen, which replicates after administration to induce an immune response.

Recombinant vaccines consist of genetically engineered antigens, which are typically inactivated, but can occasionally be live-attenuated.[4]

VACCINES

TETANUS, DIPHTHERIA, AND PERTUSSIS — Administration of a tetanus, diphtheria, and pertussis vaccine has been part of routine childhood immunization since the 1940s. For many years, however, adults were revaccinated only with inactivated adsorbed tetanus and diphtheria toxoids (Td) vaccine because of concerns about reactions to the previously used whole-cell pertussis vaccine. Two vaccines containing tetanus and diphtheria toxoids combined with protein components of acellular pertussis (Tdap; *Adacel, Boostrix*) were introduced in 2005 as a booster for adults.[5]

Pertussis infection can occur when vaccine-induced immunity has waned over time. Infected parents and siblings have transmitted pertussis to unimmunized and underimmunized infants.

Recommendations for Use – Adults with an uncertain history of primary vaccination should receive 3 doses of a Td-containing vaccine, one of which (preferably the first) should be Tdap. The first 2 doses should be administered at least 4 weeks apart and the third dose 6-12 months after the second. A Td booster should be given every 10 years. Any adult who has never received a dose of Tdap should receive one as soon as possible, regardless of the interval since the last Td-containing vaccine.

Pregnant women should receive Tdap during each pregnancy, regardless of the interval since the last Td or Tdap vaccination, to protect the newborn against pertussis in the first months of life. The vaccine should be given during the early part of gestational weeks 27 through 36 to maximize the transfer of maternal antibodies closer to birth.[6,7] Pregnant women with an uncertain or incomplete history of primary vaccination should be given 3 doses of a Td-containing vaccine, one of which should be Tdap. Women who have never received Tdap and did not receive it during pregnancy should be vaccinated immediately postpartum.

Adverse Effects – Injection-site reactions are common with administration of Td or Tdap, but they are usually mild. Fever and injection-site pain have been more frequent with Tdap than with Td. Arthus-type reactions with extensive painful swelling can occur in adults with a history of repeated vaccinations.

MEASLES, MUMPS, AND RUBELLA (MMR) — In the US, routine vaccination of children has eliminated endemic transmission of measles and rubella, and has almost eliminated mumps. Recent increases in measles cases in Europe and Southeast Asia have led to increases in imported measles cases in the US; these cases have occurred primarily in unvaccinated persons.[8] Sporadic mumps outbreaks also continue to occur, even among highly vaccinated groups.[9]

The MMR vaccine contains live-attenuated viruses; measles and mumps viruses are both derived from chick embryo cell culture and rubella virus is derived from human diploid cell culture.

Recommendations for Use – Adults born in the US before 1957 (1970 in Canada) can be considered immune to measles, mumps, and rubella. Most other adults who lack evidence of immunity (documentation of vaccination or laboratory evidence of immunity) should receive one dose of MMR. Two doses of the vaccine, separated by at least 28 days, are recommended for adults previously vaccinated with the killed (or an unknown) measles vaccine used from 1963 to 1967 and for those without evidence of immunity who are at high risk of exposure to or transmission of measles or mumps, including students in postsecondary educational institutions, international travelers, and household contacts of immunocompromised persons.[10] Healthcare workers born during or after 1957 who do not have evidence of immunity to measles and/or mumps should receive 2 doses of MMR vaccine; those who have evidence of

3

Table 1. Some Vaccines for Adults

Vaccines	Usual Dose/Schedule
Tetanus, Diphtheria (Td)	
Tetanus and diphtheria toxoids[3] Tenivac (Sanofi Pasteur)[3]	0.5 mL IM/3 doses (0, 1, and 6-12 mos)
Tetanus, Diphtheria, Acellular Pertussis (Tdap)	
Adacel (Sanofi Pasteur)[3] Boostrix (GSK)[3]	0.5 mL IM/1 lifetime booster dose[4]
Measles, Mumps, Rubella (MMR)	
M-M-R II (Merck)[6]	0.5 mL SC/1 or 2 doses[7]
Varicella (VAR)	
Varivax (Merck)[6]	0.5 mL SC/2 doses (0, 4-8 wks)
Zoster	
Shingrix (RZV; GSK)[3] Zostavax (ZVL; Merck)[6]	0.5 mL IM/2 doses (0, 2-6 mos) 0.65 mL SC/1 dose
Human Papillomavirus (HPV)	
Gardasil 9 (Merck)[3]	0.5 mL IM/3 doses (0, 1-2, and 6 mos)[9,10]

1. Based on ACIP-recommended age ranges, which may differ from FDA-approved age ranges for some vaccines. See Table 2 for vaccination of special populations. See text for detailed information on indications, contraindications, and risk factors.
2. Approximate private sector cost (including excise tax) for 1 dose as of April 1, 2018, according to the CDC Vaccine Price List. Available at: www.cdc.gov/vaccines/programs/vfc/awardees/vaccine-management/price-list/index.html?s_cid=cs_000. Accessed April 26, 2018.
3. Inactivated vaccine.
4. Pregnant women should receive Tdap during each pregnancy, ideally during the early part of gestational weeks 27-36.
5. Although Adacel is not FDA-approved for persons ≥65 years old, the ACIP recommends use of either Boostrix or Adacel in persons ≥65 years old.

Recommendations[1]	Cost[2]
▸ Primary series recommended for previously unvaccinated adults	$23.90
▸ Booster dose recommended every 10 years	32.90
▸ Single dose recommended for adults who have never received a Tdap vaccine regardless of interval since last Td[5]	44.20 40.10
▸ Recommended for adults born during or after 1957 (1970 in Canada) without evidence of immunity	70.90
▸ Recommended for adults born during or after 1980 without evidence of immunity	122.00
▸ RZV is recommended for adults ≥50 years old including those with a previous episode of herpes zoster or previous use of ZVL[8] ▸ RZV or ZVL is recommended (RZV is preferred) for adults ≥60 years old, including those with a previous episode of herpes zoster	140.00 212.70
▸ Recommended for previously unvaccinated females through age 26 years and males through age 21 years, and males 22-26 years old with risk factors or based on individual clinical decision	204.90

6. Live-attenuated vaccine.
7. One to 2 doses for no evidence of immunity to measles and mumps (second dose must be administered at least 28 days after the first) and 1 dose for no evidence of immunity to rubella. One additional dose is recommended for adults who previously received ≤2 doses and are at risk for acquiring mumps because of an outbreak.
8. RZV should not be administered <2 months after ZVL.
9. Minimum interval between doses 1 and 2 is 4 weeks, between doses 2 and 3 is 12 weeks, and between doses 1 and 3 is 5 months.
10. A 3-dose series is recommended for previously unvaccinated persons 15-26 years old. For those who started a series at age 9-14 years, but only received 1 dose or 2 doses <5 months apart, 1 additional dose is recommended.

Continued on next page

Table 1. Some Vaccines for Adults (continued)

Vaccines	Usual Dose/Schedule
Pneumococcal	
Prevnar 13 (PCV13; Pfizer)[3]	0.5 mL IM/1 dose
Pneumovax 23 (PPSV23; Merck)[3]	0.5 mL IM or SC/1-3 doses[13]
Hepatitis A (HepA)	
Havrix (GSK)[3]	1 mL IM/2 doses (0 and 6-12 mos)
Vaqta (Merck)[3]	1 mL IM/2 doses (0 and 6-18 mos)
Hepatitis B (HepB)	
Heplisav-B (Dynavax)[3]	0.5 mL IM/2 doses (0 and 1 mo)
Engerix-B (GSK)[3]	1 mL IM/3 doses (0, 1, and 6 mos)[15-17]
Recombivax HB (Merck)[3]	1 mL IM/3 doses (0, 1, and 6 mos)[15,17]
Hepatitis A/B (HepA/HepB)	
Twinrix (GSK)[3]	1 mL IM/3 doses (0, 1, and 6 mos)[19]

11. When both vaccines are indicated, PCV13 should be given first. (See pages 16-17 for information on indications and timing).
12. Risk factors include immunodeficiency disorders, HIV infection, asplenia, chronic renal failure and nephrotic syndrome, cerebrospinal fluid leak, and cochlear implants (see Table 3).
13. Adults <65 years old with risk factors should receive 1 dose or 2 doses at least 5 years apart. Adults ≥65 years old should receive 1 dose, regardless of previous vaccination history, but at least 5 years after the last PPSV23 dose.
14. Risk factors include chronic heart, lung, or liver disease, alcoholism, diabetes, cigarette smoking, immunodeficiency disorders, HIV infection, asplenia, chronic renal failure and nephrotic syndrome, cerebrospinal fluid leak, and cochlear implants (see Table 3).
15. Dose of *Engerix-B* for hemodialysis is 2 mL given at 0, 1, 2, and 6 months. *Recombivax HB* has a separate dialysis formulation (40 mcg in 1 mL) given at 0, 1, and 6 months. This dosing schedule can also be considered for immunocompromised persons.

Recommendations[1]	Cost[2]
▶ PCV13 is recommended for previously unvaccinated adults ≥65 years old and for those <65 years old with specific risk factors[11,12] ▶ PPSV23 is recommended for adults ≥65 years old (1 dose) and for those <65 years old with specific risk factors (1-2 doses)[11,14]	$94.50 180.10
▶ Recommended for previously unvaccinated adults with medical, occupational, or behavioral risk factors ▶ Recommended for adults who lack a risk factor but want protection	65.70 66.90
▶ Recommended for previously unvaccinated adults with medical, occupational, or behavioral risk factors ▶ Recommended for adults who lack a risk factor but want protection	115.00 55.70 60.50[18]
▶ Recommended for adults who require both HepA and HepB vaccine ▶ Recommended for adults who lack a risk factor but want protection	101.00

16. A 4-dose schedule at 0, 1, 2, and 12 months is also FDA-approved.
17. Alternative vaccination schedules (0, 1, and 4 months or 0, 2, and 4 months) are also recommended by ACIP. The minimum interval between doses 1 and 2 is 4 weeks, between doses 2 and 3 is 8 weeks, and between doses 1 and 3 is 16 weeks.
18. Approximate WAC for 1 dose. WAC = wholesaler acquisition cost or manufacturer's published price to wholesalers; WAC represents a published catalogue or list price and may not represent an actual transactional price. Source: AnalySource® Monthly. April 5, 2018. Reprinted with permission by First Databank, Inc. All rights reserved. ©2018. www.fdbhealth.com/policies/drug-pricing-policy.
19. The minimum interval between doses 1 and 2 is 4 weeks and between doses 2 and 3 is 5 months. A 4-dose accelerated schedule at 0, 7, 21-30 days, and 12 months is also FDA-approved.

Continued on next page

Table 1. Some Vaccines for Adults (continued)

Vaccines	Usual Dose/Schedule
Meningococcal	
Serogroups ACWY (MenACWY)	
Menveo (Novartis)[3]	0.5 mL IM/1-2 doses[20,21]
Menactra (Sanofi Pasteur)[3]	0.5 mL IM/1-2 doses[20,21]
Serogroup B (MenB)	
Bexsero (GSK)[3,22]	0.5 mL IM/2 doses (≥1 mo apart)
Trumenba (Pfizer)[3,22]	0.5 mL IM/2 or 3 doses[23]
***Haemophilus influenzae* type b (Hib)**	
ActHIB (Sanofi Pasteur)[3]	0.5 mL IM/1 or 3 doses[24]
PedvaxHIB (Merck)[3]	
Hiberix (GSK)[3]	

20. Two doses given ≥8 weeks apart are recommended for adults with asplenia, HIV infection, persistent complement component deficiencies, or eculizumab *(Soliris)* use. One dose is recommended for those with other specific risk factors.
21. Revaccination every 5 years is recommended for those previously vaccinated who remain at high risk.
22. Bexsero and Trumenba are not interchangeable.
23. Healthy young adults 16-23 years old not at increased risk for meningococcal disease may receive a 2-dose series (0 and 6 months). Those with specific risk factors should receive a 3-dose series (0, 1-2, and 6 months).

immunity to mumps and measles, but not to rubella should receive one dose. MMR vaccination should be considered for healthcare workers born before 1957 if they do not have evidence of immunity to measles, mumps, and rubella. For control of a mumps outbreak in a setting with intense exposure, high attack rates, and evidence of ongoing transmission, one additional dose of MMR vaccine is recommended for those who previously received ≤2 doses.[11]

One dose of MMR vaccine should be administered to nonpregnant women of childbearing age who lack evidence of immunity to rubella. **Pregnant women** should not receive MMR vaccine; those who do not have evidence of immunity to rubella should receive MMR vaccine postpartum, before discharge from the healthcare facility.

Recommendations[1]	Cost[2]
► Recommended for previously unvaccinated adults with specific risk factors	$127.00
	116.30
► Recommended for adults with specific risk factors; may administer to persons 16-23 years old (preferred age 16-18 years) not at increased risk	165.80
	133.60
► Recommended only for a small number of previously unvaccinated adults with specific risk factors	16.10
	26.20
	10.60

24. One dose for unimmunized asplenic persons and those undergoing elective splenectomy. Three doses (at least 4 weeks apart) for all recipients of hematopoietic stem cell transplants (beginning 6-12 months after transplant), even if previously vaccinated.

Adverse Effects – Pain and erythema at the injection site, fever, rash, and transient arthralgias (in about 25% of women) are common following MMR vaccination. Few adverse events have been reported after a third dose of MMR vaccine. Anaphylactic reactions and thrombocytopenic purpura occur rarely.[10]

Contraindications – Because MMR is a live vaccine, it is contraindicated in **pregnant women** (the risk of congenital rubella syndrome from the vaccine may be only theoretical; it has not been reported among the thousands of infants born to women vaccinated inadvertently during pregnancy) and in adults with severe immunodeficiency. The vaccine should not be given to persons with a history of anaphylaxis caused by neomycin or gelatin.

VARICELLA — The varicella vaccine contains live-attenuated varicella virus. Routine childhood immunization, introduced in the US in 1995, has resulted in a sharp decline in the incidence of varicella infection in both children and adults. Primary varicella infection can be more severe in adults than in children.

Recommendations for Use – Persons born in the US before 1980 are considered immune to varicella, except for healthcare workers and pregnant women, who should be evaluated for evidence of immunity. Evidence of immunity to varicella is demonstrated by: a history of varicella or herpes zoster diagnosed by a healthcare provider, laboratory evidence of immunity (not always reliable), or documentation of vaccination. Adult immigrants newly arrived in the US from tropical countries may be susceptible to varicella. All adults without evidence of immunity should receive 2 doses of vaccine at least 4 weeks apart. Nonimmune **pregnant women** should receive the first dose postpartum before discharge from the healthcare facility.[12] Immunity after vaccination is probably permanent in the majority of vaccinees.

Adverse Effects – Injection-site reactions such as soreness, erythema, and swelling are common in adults. Other adverse effects include fever and varicella-like rash (at the injection site or generalized, usually occurring within 2-3 weeks after vaccination). Spread of vaccine virus from healthy vaccinees who develop a varicella-like rash to susceptible contacts is rare. Recipients who have a vaccine-related rash should avoid contact with susceptible individuals who are at high risk of varicella complications, such as immunocompromised persons, pregnant women, and neonates born to nonimmune mothers.

Contraindications – Because it is a live vaccine, varicella vaccine is contraindicated in **pregnant women** and in persons with severe immunodeficiency. It should not be given to persons with a history of anaphylaxis caused by neomycin or gelatin.

ZOSTER — Following resolution of a primary infection, varicella-zoster virus (VZV) persists in a latent form in sensory ganglia; VZV-specific cell-mediated immunity (CMI) prevents latent virus from reactivating and multiplying to cause herpes zoster. When CMI declines, as it can in older persons and those who are immunocompromised, latent VZV can reactivate and cause herpes zoster ("shingles"). About 1 million cases of shingles occur in the US every year.

Two different zoster vaccines are now FDA-licensed for use in the US: a live-attenuated vaccine (ZVL; *Zostavax*) and a new adjuvanted recombinant subunit vaccine (RZV; *Shingrix*).[13] In randomized, double-blind clinical trials, ZVL significantly reduced the incidence of herpes zoster in adults 50-79 years old, but not in those ≥80 years old; its effectiveness declined sharply with age (70% at ages 50-59 years, 64% at 60-69 years, 41% at 70-79 years, 18% at ≥80 years).[14,15] In a large cohort study in adults ≥50 years old, ZVL was about 68% effective in preventing herpes zoster in the first year after vaccination; efficacy decreased to 47% in the second year, and continued to decline gradually over the next 6 years to 32%.[16]

Although no direct comparisons are available, RZV appears to be considerably more effective than ZVL in preventing herpes zoster. In observer-blinded clinical trials in >27,000 persons, RZV was highly effective in preventing herpes zoster in all age groups, especially older persons (97% in those 50-59 and 60-69 years old and 91% in those 70-79 and ≥80 years old). The duration of protection with RZV is unknown; in persons ≥70 years old, vaccine efficacy was 85.1% in the fourth year after vaccination.[17,18]

Recommendations for Use – Immunocompetent adults ≥50 years old, including those with a history of herpes zoster and those who have already received ZVL, should be vaccinated with two doses of RZV (2-6 months apart). RZV should not be given <2 months after vaccination

Table 2. Adult Vaccines for Special Populations*

Risk Groups	HPV	Td/Tdap	Influenza	Pneumococcal
Pregnancy	NR	✓[1]	✓[2]	NR[3]
Immunocompromising conditions[6,7] (except HIV)	✓	✓	✓[2]	✓
Diabetes	✓	✓	✓[2]	✓[11]
Cardiac or pulmonary[13] disease, or chronic alcoholism	✓	✓	✓	✓[11]
Asplenia,[14] complement deficiencies (including eculizumab use)	✓	✓	✓[2,15]	✓
End-stage kidney disease (including hemodialysis)	✓	✓	✓[2]	✓
Chronic liver disease	✓	✓	✓[2]	✓[11]
HIV[6]				
CD4 count <200 cells/mcL	✓	✓	✓[2]	✓
CD4 count >200 cells/mcL	✓	✓	✓[2]	✓
Healthcare workers	✓	✓	✓	RF
Men who have sex with men	✓	✓	✓	RF

*See Table 1 for age restrictions
✓ = recommended; RF = recommended if another risk factor is present; X = contraindicated;
NR = no recommendation; RZV = recombinant zoster vaccine; ZVL = zoster vaccine live
1. Women should receive Tdap during each pregnancy, preferably during the early part of gestational weeks 27 through 36.
2. Only inactivated influenza vaccine is recommended.
3. For PCV13, no recommendation has been published. For PPSV23, insufficient data for specific recommendation; no adverse effects have been reported in newborns whose mothers were vaccinated during pregnancy.
4. Pregnant women who are not immune to rubella and/or varicella should receive one dose of MMR vaccine and/or varicella vaccine after delivery and before discharge from the healthcare facility. The second dose of varicella should be given 4-8 weeks after the first dose.
5. MenACWY may be used if otherwise indicated. For MenB, base decision on risk vs benefit.
6. See also published guidelines for vaccination of immunocompromised hosts (LG Rubin et al. Clin Infect Dis 2014; 58:e44; M Tomblyn et al. Biol Blood Marrow Transplant 2009; 15:1143).
7. If possible, indicated vaccines should be given before starting chemotherapy, treatment with other immunosuppressive drugs, or radiation.
8. Persons with leukemia, lymphoma, or other malignancies in remission with no recent history (≥3 months) of chemotherapy are not considered severely immunosuppressed for the purpose of receiving live-virus vaccines.
9. Wait at least 1 month after discontinuing long-term administration of high-dose corticosteroids before giving a live-virus vaccine. The definition of high-dose or long-term corticosteroids is considered by most clinicians to be ≥20 mg/day of prednisone or its equivalent for ≥14 days. Short-term (<2 weeks) treatment, low to moderate doses, long-term alternate-day treatment with short-acting preparations, maintenance physiologic doses (replacement therapy), or steroids administered topically, by aerosol, or by intra-articular, bursal, or tendon injection are not considered contraindications to live-virus vaccines.

MMR	Vari-cella	Zoster RZV	Zoster ZVL	Hep B	Hep A	Meningo-coccal	Hib
X[4]	X[4]	NR	X	RF	RF	RF[5]	NR
X[8,9]	X[8,9]	NR	X[8,9]	RF	RF	RF	✓[10]
✓	✓	✓	✓	✓[12]	RF	RF	RF
✓	✓	✓	✓	RF	RF	RF	RF
✓	✓	✓	✓	RF	RF	✓	✓[16]
✓	✓	✓	✓	✓[17]	RF	RF	RF
✓	✓	✓	✓	✓	✓	RF	RF
X	X	NR	X	✓	RF	✓[18]	RF
✓	✓	NR	NR	✓	RF	✓[18]	RF
✓	✓	✓	✓	✓	RF	RF	RF
✓	✓	✓	✓	✓	✓	RF	RF

10. Recommended for hematopoietic stem cell transplant recipients only.
11. PPSV23 is recommended. PCV13 is only recommended for those with other risk factors. Cochlear implants and cerebrospinal fluid leaks are considered risk factors for both PPSV23 and PCV13.
12. Recommended for adults 19-59 years old, and may be considered for those ≥60 years old based on individual clinical decision.
13. Chronic pulmonary diseases include chronic pneumonitis, chronic obstructive pulmonary disease, chronic bronchitis, or asthma.
14. Functional or anatomic asplenia, including elective splenectomy. When possible, persons undergoing elective splenectomy should receive the indicated vaccines ≥2 weeks before surgery.
15. No data exist on the risk for severe or complicated influenza in persons with asplenia. However, influenza is a risk factor for secondary bacterial infections that can be life-threatening in asplenic patients.
16. Only recommended for those who never received a primary series and a booster dose at age ≥12 months or at least 1 dose after the age of 14 months.
17. For adults on hemodialysis the dosage of *Engerix-B* is 2 mL given at 0, 1, 2, and 6 months, and the dosage of *Recombivax HB* is 40 mcg/1 mL (dialysis formulation) given at 0, 1, and 6 months. No dosage has been defined for *Heplisav-B*.
18. MenACWY is recommended. MenB is only recommended for those with other indications.

with ZVL. RZV is preferred over ZVL, but ZVL remains an alternative for immunocompetent adults ≥60 years old.[19]

Adverse Effects – Adverse reactions appear to be more frequent and more severe with RZV than with ZVL. Common adverse effects of RZV include myalgia (45%), fatigue (45%), fever (21%), and injection-site pain (78%), redness (38%), and swelling (26%). In clinical trials with RZV, the incidence of any grade 3 adverse event was 16.5% and the incidence of grade 3 injection-site reactions was 9.4%; the median duration of local and systemic adverse effects was 2-3 days. Injection-site reactions with ZVL are generally mild; varicella-like rash has occurred at the injection site, but is less common than with varicella vaccination.

Contraindications – Because it is a live vaccine, ZVL is contraindicated in **pregnant women** and in adults with severe immunodeficiency. It should not be given to persons with a history of an anaphylactic reaction to neomycin or gelatin. RZV is not contraindicated in pregnant women and immunocompromised adults, but its safety and efficacy in these populations have not yet been established.

HUMAN PAPILLOMAVIRUS (HPV) — HPV is a common sexually transmitted infection often acquired soon after initiation of sexual activity. Although most HPV infections clear spontaneously without clinical sequelae, persistent infection with an oncogenic HPV type can cause abnormalities in the cervical epithelium that may progress to cancer. Oncogenic HPV types 16 and 18 cause about 70% of cervical cancers and about 80% of anal cancers. Non-oncogenic types 6 and 11 cause 90% of genital warts. Five additional HPV types, 31, 33, 45, 52, and 58, are responsible for an additional 15% of cervical cancers. These HPV types are also associated with non-anogenital cancers, particularly oropharyngeal cancers.

A recombinant 9-valent vaccine *(Gardasil 9)* is the only HPV vaccine available in the US. It is licensed by the FDA for use in both men and women to prevent diseases associated with HPV types 6, 11, 16, 18, 31, 33,

45, 52, and 58, including genital warts and cervical, vulvar, vaginal, and anal precancerous lesions and cancer.[20,21] The bivalent vaccine *(Cervarix)*, which protected against HPV types 16 and 18, and the quadrivalent vaccine *(Gardasil)*, which protected against HPV types 6, 11, 16, and 18, have been discontinued. Compared to the quadrivalent vaccine, the 9-valent vaccine reduced the risk of high-grade cervical, vulvar, or vaginal disease related to HPV types 31, 33, 45, 52, or 58 by 97%; antibody responses to the 4 HPV types found in both vaccines were similar, as was the incidence of disease or persistent infection related to those HPV types.[22]

Recommendations for Use – Routine HPV vaccination is recommended for girls and boys 11-12 years old (can start at age 9). Previously unvaccinated females 15 through 26 years old and males 15 through 21 years old should receive a 3-dose series (0, 1-2, and 6 months); a 2-dose schedule (0 and 6-12 months) is recommended for those who start the series before their 15th birthday. Adults who received 1 dose or 2 doses <5 months apart before age 15 years should receive 1 additional dose. Transgender persons and men who have sex with men should be vaccinated through age 26 with a 2- or 3-dose series depending on the age at which they start the series. Immunocompromised females and males are at higher risk for HPV infection and should be vaccinated with a 3-dose series through age 26.[21,23]

Although the vaccine should ideally be administered before the onset of sexual activity, persons ≤26 years old who have already been exposed to HPV or diagnosed with HPV infection (based on an abnormal Pap smear or presence of genital warts) should also be vaccinated because they may not have been exposed to all the HPV types included in the vaccine. A schedule started with the bivalent or quadrivalent vaccine can be completed with the 9-valent vaccine. The duration of immunity is not known, but it appears to be at least 8-10 years; booster doses are not currently recommended.

HPV vaccine is not recommended for **pregnant women** due to limited data; no increase in adverse outcomes was reported among women exposed to the quadrivalent vaccine during the periconceptional period or during pregnancy.[24,25]

Adverse Effects – Injection-site reactions such as pain, swelling, and erythema can occur. Syncope has been reported; patients should be seated or lying down during vaccine administration and observed for 15 minutes afterwards.

PNEUMOCOCCAL — Adults with immunocompromising conditions and those ≥65 years old have an increased risk of developing invasive pneumococcal disease. Routine childhood immunization has resulted in a 90% reduction in vaccine-type invasive pneumococcal disease and a 50% reduction in overall disease.

Two pneumococcal vaccines are FDA-licensed for use in adults, a conjugate vaccine that contains 13 serotypes of pneumococcus (PCV13; *Prevnar 13*)[26] and a 23-valent pneumococcal polysaccharide vaccine (PPSV23; *Pneumovax 23*). The pneumococcal serotypes in PCV13 cause about half of the cases of invasive pneumococcal disease in immunocompromised adults; an additional one-fifth are caused by serotypes contained only in PPSV23. In a placebo-controlled trial in nearly 85,000 adults ≥65 years old (CAPITA), vaccination with PCV13 reduced first episodes of vaccine-type nonbacteremic and noninvasive community-acquired pneumonia and invasive pneumococcal disease by 45% and 75%, respectively.[27]

The serotypes in PPSV23 cause 60-76% of bacteremic pneumococcal disease.[28] The vaccine is effective in preventing invasive disease, but randomized controlled trials and cohort studies in the general population and in those ≥65 years old have not consistently shown that it decreases the incidence of noninvasive pneumococcal pneumonia, and its protective effect appears to wane after 5 years.[29-31]

Recommendations for Use – All adults ≥65 years old should receive a one-time dose of PCV13 and one dose of PPSV23. For those who

Table 3. Recommendations for Pneumococcal Vaccination
All Adults ≥65 years old
PCV13 x 1 dose[1], then PPSV23 ≥1 year later[2]
Adults <65 years old who smoke cigarettes or have diabetes, alcohol use disorder, or chronic lung, heart, or liver disease
PPSV23 x 1 dose[3]
Adults <65 years old who have immunocompromising conditions,[4] functional or anatomic asplenia, cochlear implants, or cerebrospinal fluid leaks
PCV13 x 1 dose, then PPSV23 ≥8 weeks later[2,3,5]

1. Some Medical Letter reviewers recommend only PPSV23 for healthy adults ≥65 years old.
2. If previously vaccinated with PPSV23, PCV13 should be given at least 1 year after last dose of PPSV23.
3. All adults who received 1 or 2 doses of PPSV23 before age 65 years should be revaccinated once at age ≥65 years ≥5 years after the last PPSV23 dose.
4. HIV infection, leukemia, lymphoma, Hodgkin's disease, multiple myeloma, generalized malignancy, chronic renal failure, nephrotic syndrome, solid organ transplant, or diseases requiring treatment with immunosuppressive drugs.
5. A second dose of PPSV23 should be given to adults <65 years old with the highest risk of pneumococcal disease or rapid antibody loss, including those with immunocompromising conditions and functional or anatomic asplenia. The second PPSV23 dose should be given ≥8 weeks after PCV13, and ≥5 years after the last PPSV23 dose.

have not previously received either vaccine, PCV13 should be given first, followed at least one year later by PPSV23. Those who previously received PPSV23 should receive PCV13 at least one year after the last dose of PPSV23.[32] Some Medical Letter reviewers recommend only PPSV23 for otherwise healthy adults ≥65 years old. Recommendations for vaccination of adults who are ≥65 years old or <65 years old with specific risk factors are listed in Table 3.[33,34]

Adverse Effects – Mild to moderate injection-site reactions, headache, fatigue, and myalgia are common with PCV13 and PPSV23.

HEPATITIS A — Hepatitis A virus (HAV) infection occurs frequently in the US and is endemic in certain communities in western and southwestern states and in Alaska; the prevalence of anti-HAV antibodies ranges from about 9% in preadolescent children to about 75% in elderly adults.[4] Hepatitis A vaccine (HepA), introduced in the US in 1996, is now part of routine childhood immunization. Two inactivated hepatitis A whole-virus vaccines *(Vaqta, Havrix)* are available in the US. A combination hepatitis A and B vaccine (HepA/HepB; *Twinrix*) contains the same hepatitis A component as in *Havrix*, but half the dose.

Recommendations for Use – HepA vaccine is recommended for adults who have a medical, occupational, or behavioral risk of infection, or who lack a risk factor but want protection. Medical indications are clotting factor disorders and chronic liver disease. Occupational indications are work with HAV in a laboratory or work with HAV-infected primates. Adults with behavioral risks are illicit (injection and non-injection) drug users and men who have sex with men. HepA vaccine is also recommended for close contacts of adopted children from countries with intermediate or high rates of HAV infection, for susceptible travelers going anywhere other than Canada, Australia, New Zealand, Japan, or western Europe, and for those with recent exposure to HAV.

HepA vaccination in adults consists of 2 doses separated by at least 6 months. Antibodies reach protective levels 2-4 weeks after the first dose. The combination HepA/HepB vaccine should be given in 3 doses at 0, 1, and 6 months. HepA/HepB vaccine can also be given in an accelerated 4-dose schedule; the first 3 doses are given at 0, 7, and 21-30 days, and the fourth at 12 months. Patients who have received a first dose of one HepA vaccine can be given another one to complete the series. Booster doses are not recommended for immunocompetent adults who have completed a primary series.

Adverse Effects – Injection-site reactions such as pain, swelling, and erythema occur in about 60% of vaccine recipients. Systemic complaints such as malaise, low-grade fever, and fatigue are generally mild and occur in less than 10% of vaccinees.

HEPATITIS B — The prevalence of chronic hepatitis B virus (HBV) infection in the US is low (about 800,000-1.4 million persons). Since routine childhood immunization was introduced in 1991, the number of new cases of HBV infection has declined by 82%. In 2015, the incidence of acute HBV infection was highest among those 30-39 years old (2.6 cases/100,000 persons).[35]

All four hepatitis B vaccines (HepB) available in the US for use in adults contain recombinant yeast-derived hepatitis B surface antigen (HBsAg) with an immunostimulatory adjuvant. *Engerix-B, Recombivax HB*, and *Twinrix* (HepA/HepB vaccine) use aluminum hydroxide as an adjuvant. *Heplisav-B* uses a synthetic cytosine phosphoguanine oligonucleotide (CpG 1018) adjuvant that stimulates the immune system through activation of the toll-like receptor 9 (TLR-9) pathway.[36] *Engerix-B*, *Recombivax HB*, and *Twinrix* are usually administered in 3 doses; *Heplisav-B* is given in 2 doses.[37]

In a randomized, observer-blinded study that compared 2 doses of *Heplisav-B* to 3 doses of *Engerix-B*, seroprotection rates were significantly higher with *Heplisav-B* than with *Engerix-B* (95.4% vs 81.3%) among nearly 6500 persons 18-70 years old. Among 961 patients with diabetes, seroprotection rates were also significantly higher with *Heplisav-B* (90.0% vs 65.1%). Immune responses to both vaccines were shown to decrease with age, but seroprotection rates were significantly higher with *Heplisav-B* in all age groups.[38]

Recommendations for Use – HepB vaccination is recommended for adults who have a medical, occupational, or behavioral risk of infection, or who lack a risk factor but want protection.[39] Medical indications are end-stage renal disease (including hemodialysis), chronic liver disease, diabetes (particularly in persons 19-59 years old),[40] or HIV infection. Occupational indications include healthcare and public safety workers with potential exposure to blood or body fluids. Adults with behavioral risks include injection drug users, persons who had sex with more than one partner in the previous 6 months or recently acquired a sexually transmitted infection, and men who have sex with men.

Other populations who should receive HepB vaccine include clients of facilities that test for and treat sexually transmitted infections, HIV, or drug abuse, residents and staff of institutions for the developmentally disabled, inmates of correctional facilities, household contacts and sex partners of persons with chronic HBV infection, and travelers to countries with intermediate or high rates of chronic HBV infection. **Pregnant women** who are at risk for HBV infection during pregnancy should be vaccinated; until more data are available with *Heplisav-B*, one of the other HepB vaccines should be used.[41]

Primary immunization with *Heplisav-B* consists of 2 doses (0 and 1 month). Primary immunization with the other HepB vaccines usually consists of 3 doses (0, 1, and 6 months). An alternate schedule (0, 1, and 2 months, followed by a fourth dose at 12 months) is FDA-approved for *Engerix-B* in the US and is only intended for use in those who have recently been exposed to the virus and travelers to high-risk areas. HepA/HepB vaccine can also be given in an accelerated schedule (0, 7, and 21-30 days, followed by a fourth dose at 12 months). If possible, the same vaccine should be used for all doses of a HepB series. However, an interrupted HepB series does not have to be restarted if the same vaccine is not available. A series started with a single dose of *Engerix-B, Recombivax HB*, or *Twinrix* can be completed with 2 doses of *Heplisav-B*. One dose of *Heplisav-B* can be used as part of a 3-dose series.[41] Booster doses are not recommended for most adults who responded to primary immunization.[39]

Adverse Effects – The most common adverse effect of hepatitis B vaccination is pain at the injection site; erythema and swelling can also occur. In clinical trials, injection-site reactions were more common with *Heplisav-B* than with *Engerix-B*; rates of serious adverse events were similar with the two vaccines. Fever occurs in about 1-6% of recipients.

MENINGOCOCCAL — Fewer than 1000 cases of meningococcal disease occur in the US each year. The case fatality rate is 10-15% for meningitis and up to 40% for meningococcemia. Rates of meningococcal disease are highest in infancy. A second peak occurs in adolescents and young adults, and a third in adults ≥65 years old. *Neisseria meningitidis* serogroups B, C, and Y cause most cases of meningococcal disease in the US.

Two quadrivalent inactivated vaccines against *N. meningitidis* serogroups A, C, W, and Y (MenACWY; *Menactra, Menveo*) are available in the US. Both contain the same capsular polysaccharides.[42] In adults, both vaccines induce serogroup-specific antibody responses in more than 90% of recipients.[43] Serologic data show a significant decline in serum antibody titers 3-5 years after vaccination.[4] Neither of these vaccines provides protection against serogroup B.

Serogroup B Vaccine – In the US, serogroup B causes about 60% of all meningococcal disease in children <5 years old and about 50% of cases in young adults 17-22 years old. Several outbreaks of serogroup B meningococcal disease have occurred on college campuses in recent years.[44,45] Two serogroup B meningococcal vaccines (MenB; *Trumenba, Bexsero*), are licensed in the US for use in persons 10-25 years old.[46,47] Each contains components derived from cell surface antigens of prevalent serogroup B strains of *N. meningitidis*. They were approved based on the results of safety and immunogenicity studies. Their comparative efficacy and duration of immunity are unknown.

Recommendations for Use – Routine vaccination with **MenACWY** is recommended for adolescents 11-18 years old. Two doses given at least 8 weeks apart and one booster dose every 5 years are recommended for adults with HIV infection, functional or anatomic asplenia, or persistent complement component deficiencies (including persons taking eculizumab *[Soliris],* which impairs complement function). One dose of vaccine and revaccination every 5 years should be considered for adults who travel to or live in countries where meningococcal disease is hyperendemic or epidemic, including persons going to countries in the African meningitis belt or participating in the Hajj, persons who are at risk from a meningococcal disease outbreak attributed to serogroup A, C,

W, or Y, microbiologists routinely exposed to *N. meningitidis*, military recruits and first-year college students who live in residential housing (if they did not receive MenACWY vaccine at age 16 years or older).[48] MenACWY may be used in **pregnant women** if otherwise indicated.

MenB vaccine is recommended for adults with functional or anatomic asplenia, persons with persistent complement component deficiency or eculizumab use, those who are at risk from a meningococcal outbreak attributed to serogroup B, and microbiologists routinely exposed to *N. meningitidis*. *Bexsero* should be administered in 2 doses at least one month apart; *Trumenba* should be administered in 3 doses at 0, 1-2, and 6 months. MenB vaccine may also be considered for young adults 16 through 23 years old (preferably age 16-18 years) who are not at increased risk for serogroup B meningococcal disease; in this setting, *Trumenba* should be given in 2 doses at least 6 months apart and *Bexsero* in 2 doses one month apart.[49] The vaccines are not interchangeable; the same vaccine must be used for all doses. Either MenB vaccine may be administered concomitantly with other vaccines recommended for this age group, preferably at a different injection site. No booster doses are recommended for any group. MenB vaccination should be deferred in **pregnant women** unless the benefits are thought to outweigh the risks.

Adverse Effects – The most common adverse reactions to *Menactra* and *Menveo* are headache, fatigue, malaise, and injection-site pain, redness, and induration; rates are similar to those with tetanus toxoid. Guillian-Barré syndrome has been reported rarely in adolescents who received *Menactra*, but the risk appears to be very low (0-1.5 cases/1 million vaccines within 6 weeks after vaccination).[48]

The most common adverse effects of *Bexsero* and *Trumenba* are pain, erythema, and induration at the injection site, fatigue, headache, and myalgia.

***HAEMOPHILUS INFLUENZAE* TYPE B (Hib)** — Hib can cause bacterial meningitis and other invasive diseases. The majority of Hib disease in the US occurs in infants and children; routine vaccination of young children is recommended.[50] Three monovalent Hib conjugate vaccines (*PedvaxHIB*, *ActHIB*, and *Hiberix*) are available in the US.

Recommendations for Use – Hib vaccination is only recommended for immunocompromised adults who are considered at increased risk for invasive Hib disease.[51] A single dose of any Hib conjugate vaccine should be administered to previously unvaccinated adults who have functional or anatomic asplenia or who are scheduled for an elective splenectomy (preferably ≥14 days before the procedure). Some experts suggest administering one dose to these patients regardless of prior vaccination history. Hematopoietic stem cell transplant recipients, including those who had previously been vaccinated, should receive 3 doses of Hib vaccine (given at least 4 weeks apart) beginning 6-12 months after the transplant. Hib vaccination is not recommended for HIV-infected adults.

Adverse Effects – Hib vaccine has not been studied in adults. In children, erythema, pain, and swelling at the injection site, mild fever, irritability, vomiting, and diarrhea have occurred.

1. DK Kim et al. Advisory Committee on Immunization Practices recommended immunization schedule for adults aged 19 years or older – United States, 2018. MMWR Morb Mortal Wkly Rep 2018; 67:158.
2. Influenza vaccine for 2017-2018. Med Lett Drugs Ther 2017; 59:163.
3. Vaccines for travelers. Med Lett Drugs Ther 2014; 56:115.
4. Centers for Disease Control and Prevention (CDC). Epidemiology and prevention of vaccine-preventable diseases (The Pink Book). J Hamborsky et al. eds. 13th ed. Washington D.C. Public Health Foundation, 2015. Available at: www.cdc.gov/vaccines/pubs/pinkbook/index.html. Accessed April 26, 2018.
5. Adacel and Boostrix: Tdap vaccines for adolescents and adults. Med Lett Drugs Ther 2006; 48:5.
6. Centers for Disease Control and Prevention (CDC). Updated recommendations for use of tetanus toxoid, reduced diphtheria toxoid, and acellular pertussis vaccine (Tdap) in pregnant women – Advisory Committee on Immunization Practices (ACIP), 2012. MMWR Morb Mortal Wkly Rep 2013; 62:131.
7. Centers for Disease Control and Prevention (CDC). ACIP Meeting Summary Report, October 2016. Available at: www.cdc.gov/vaccines/acip/meetings/downloads/min-archive/min-2016-10.pdf. Accessed April 26, 2018.

8. Centers for Disease Control and Prevention. Measles – United States, January 1-May 3, 2014. MMWR Morb Mortal Wkly Rep 2014; 63:496.

9. JP Albertson et al. Mumps outbeak at a university and recommendation for a third dose of measles-mumps-rubella vaccine—Illinois, 2015-2016. MMWR Morb Mortal Wkly Rep 2016; 65:731.

10. HQ McLean et al. Prevention of measles, rubella, congenital rubella syndrome, and mumps, 2013: summary recommendations of the Advisory Committee on Immunization Practices (ACIP). MMWR Recomm Rep 2013; 62(RR-4):1.

11. M Marin et al. Recommendation of the Advisory Committee on Immunization Practices for use of a third dose of mumps virus-containing vaccine in persons at increased risk for mumps during an outbreak. MMWR Morbid Mortal Wkly Rep 2018; 67:33.

12. M Marin et al. Prevention of varicella: recommendations of the Advisory Committee on Immunization Practices (ACIP). MMWR Recomm Rep 2007; 56 (RR-4):1.

13. Shingrix – an adjuvanted, recombinant herpes zoster vaccine. Med Lett Drugs Ther 2017; 59:195.

14. MN Oxman et al. A vaccine to prevent herpes zoster and postherpetic neuralgia in older adults. N Engl J Med 2005; 352:2271.

15. KE Schmader et al. Efficacy, safety, and tolerability of herpes zoster vaccine in persons aged 50-59 years. Clin Infect Dis 2012; 54:922.

16. R Baxter et al. Long-term effectiveness of the live zoster vaccine in preventing shingles: a cohort study. Am J Epidemiol 2018; 187:161.

17. H Lal et al. Efficacy of an adjuvanted herpes zoster subunit vaccine in older adults. N Engl J Med 2015; 372:2087.

18. AL Cunningham et al. Efficacy of the herpes zoster subunit vaccine in adults 70 years of age or older. N Engl J Med 2016; 375:1019.

19. KL Dooling et al. Recommendations of the Advisory Committee on Immunization Practices for use of herpes zoster vaccines. MMWR Morb Mortal Wkly Rep 2018; 67:103.

20. Gardasil 9 - a broader HPV vaccine. Med Lett Drugs Ther 2015; 57:47.

21. E Petrosky et al. Use of 9-valent human papillomavirus (HPV) vaccine: updated HPV vaccination recommendations of the Advisory Committee on Immunization Practices. MMWR Morb Mortal Wkly Rep 2015; 64:300.

22. WK Huh et al. Final efficacy, immunogenicity, and safety analyses of a nine-valent human papillomavirus vaccine in women aged 16-26 years: a randomised, double-blind trial. Lancet 2017; 390:2143.

23. E Meites et al. Use of a 2-dose schedule for human papillomavirus (HPV) vaccination – updated recommendations of the Advisory Committee on Immunization Practices. MMWR Morb Mortal Wkly Rep 2016; 65:1405.

24. NM Scheller et al. Quadrivalent HPV vaccination and the risk of adverse pregnancy outcomes. N Engl J Med 2017; 376:1223.

25. HS Lipkind et al. Maternal and infant outcomes after human papillomavirus vaccination in the periconceptional period or during pregnancy. Obstet Gynecol 2017; 130:599.

26. Pneumococcal vaccine for adults. Med Lett Drugs Ther 2012; 54:87.

27. MJ Bonten et al. Polysaccharide conjugate vaccine against pneumococcal pneumonia in adults. N Engl J Med 2015; 372:1114.

28. Centers for Disease Control and Prevention (CDC) and Advisory Committee on Immunization Practices. Updated recommendations for prevention of invasive pneumococcal disease among adults using the 23-valent pneumococcal polysaccharide vaccine (PPSV23). MMWR Morb Mortal Wkly Rep 2010; 59:1102.

29. G Falkenhorst et al. Effectiveness of the 23-valent pneumococcal polysaccharide vaccine (PPV23) against pneumococcal disease in the elderly: systematic review and meta-analysis. PLoS One 2017; 12:e0169368.

30. O Ochoa-Gondar et al. Effectiveness of the 23-valent pneumococcal polysaccharide vaccine against community-acquired pneumonia in the general population age ≥60 years: 3 years of follow-up in the CAPAMIS study. Clin Infect Dis 2014; 58:909.

31. M Suzuki et al. Serotype-specific effectiveness of 23-valent pneumococcal polysaccharide vaccine against pneumococcal pneumonia in adults aged 65 years or older: a multicenter, prospective, test-negative design study. Lancet Infect Dis 2017; 17:313.

32. M Kobayashi et al. Intervals between PCV13 and PPSV23 vaccines: recommendations of the Advisory Committee on Immunization Practices (ACIP). MMWR Morb Mortal Wkly Rep 2015; 64:944.

33. Centers for Disease Control and Prevention (CDC). Use of 13-valent pneumococcal conjugate vaccine and 23-valent pneumococcal polysaccharide vaccine for adults with immunocompromising conditions: recommendations of the Advisory Committee on Immunization Practices (ACIP). MMWR Morb Mortal Wkly Rep 2012; 61:816.

34. Centers for Disease Control and Prevention (CDC). Pneumococcal vaccine timing for adults. November 30, 2015. Available at: www.cdc.gov/vaccines/vpd/pneumo/downloads/pneumo-vaccine-timing.pdf. Accessed April 26, 2018.

35. Centers for Disease Control and Prevention (CDC). Surveillance for viral hepatitis – United States, 2015. Available at: www.cdc.gov/hepatitis/statistics/2015surveillance/index.htm. Accessed April 26, 2018.

36. NF Eng et al. The potential of 1018 ISS adjuvant in hepatitis B vaccines: Heplisav™ review. Hum Vaccin Immunother 2013; 9:1661.

37. A two-dose hepatitis B vaccine for adults (Heplisav-B). Med Lett Drugs Ther 2018; 60:17.

38. S Jackson et al. Immunogenicity of a two-dose investigational hepatitis B vaccine, HBsAg-1018, using a toll-like receptor 9 agonist adjuvant compared with a licensed hepatitis B vaccine in adults. Vaccine 2018; 36:668.

39. Centers for Disease Control and Prevention (CDC). Prevention of hepatitis B virus infection in the United States: recommendations of the Advisory Committee on Immunization Practices. MMWR Recomm Rep 2018; 67(RR-1):1.

40. Centers for Disease Control and Prevention (CDC). Use of hepatitis B vaccination for adults with diabetes mellitus: recommendations of the Advisory Committee on Immunization Practices (ACIP). MMWR Morb Mortal Wkly Rep 2011; 60:1709.

41. S Schillie et al. Recommendations of the Advisory Committee on Immunization Practices for use of a hepatitis B vaccine with a novel adjuvant. MMWR Morb Mortal Wkly Rep 2018; 67:455.

42. A new conjugate meningococcal vaccine (Menveo). Med Lett Drugs Ther 2010; 52:59.

43. KS Reisinger et al. Quadrivalent meningococcal vaccination of adults: phase III comparison of an investigational conjugate vaccine, MenACWY-CRM, with the licensed vaccine, Menactra. Clin Vaccine Immunol 2009; 16:1810.

44. HM Soeters et al. Serogroup B meningococcal disease outbreak and carriage evaluation at a college – Rhode Island, 2015. MMWR Morb Mortal Wkly Rep 2015; 64:606.

45. LA McNamara et al. First use of serogroup B meningococcal vaccine in the US in response to a university outbreak. Pediatrics 2015; 135:798.

46. Bexsero – a second serogroup B meningococcal vaccine. Med Lett Drugs Ther 2015; 57:158.

47. Trumenba: a serogroup B meningococcal vaccine. Med Lett Drugs Ther 2015; 57:5.

48. AC Cohn et al. Prevention and control of meningococcal disease: recommendations of the Advisory Committee on Immunization Practices (ACIP). MMWR Recomm Rep 2013; 62(RR-2):1.

49. T Folaranmi et al. Use of serogroup B meningococcal vaccines in persons aged ≥10 years at increased risk for serogroup B meningococcal disease: recommendations of the Advisory Committee on Immunization Practices, 2015. MMWR Morb Mortal Wkly Rep 2015; 64:608.

50. HM Soeters et al. Current epidemiology and trends in invasive Haemophilus influenzae disease–United States, 2009-2015. Clin Infect Dis 2018 March 2 (epub).

51. EC Briere et al. Prevention and control of Haemophilus influenzae type b disease: recommendations of the Advisory Committee on Immunization Practices (ACIP). MMWR Recomm Rep 2014; 63(RR-1):1.

DRUGS FOR
Rheumatoid Arthritis

Original publication date – July 2018

CONVENTIONAL DMARDs

Disease-modifying antirheumatic drugs (DMARDs) are used for initial treatment of rheumatoid arthritis (RA) to achieve clinical remission and prevent irreversible joint damage (see Table 1).[1] DMARDs generally do not have an immediate analgesic effect, but over time they can control symptoms and have been shown to delay and possibly stop progression of the disease. Methotrexate (*Trexall,* and others) is generally the drug of choice; it can be used for patients with low, moderate, or high disease activity. For mild disease, some clinicians prefer to start with hydroxychloroquine (*Plaquenil*, and generics) and/or sulfasalazine (*Azulfidine*, and others).

METHOTREXATE — Even in low doses, methotrexate can decrease symptoms, limit joint damage, and improve outcomes. The antirheumatic effect of methotrexate usually becomes apparent within 3-6 weeks of starting treatment, but sometimes it can take several months. Renal toxicity is more likely to occur in patients with renal impairment; the drug is not recommended for patients with a CrCl <30 mL/min. Methotrexate should generally not be used in patients with pre-existing liver disease or in those who consume large amounts of alcohol. Hepatic transaminase levels should be monitored before and during treatment. Patients should be screened for active hepatitis B and C infection before starting the drug.

Recommendations for Treatment of Rheumatoid Arthritis

▸ A disease-modifying antirheumatic drug (DMARD) should be used for initial treatment of rheumatoid arthritis (RA).

▸ Methotrexate is generally the DMARD of choice for patients with low, moderate, or high disease activity, but hydroxychloroquine and/or sulfasalazine can be used for mild disease.

▸ A nonsteroidal anti-inflammatory drug (NSAID) or corticosteroid can be used for symptom control until DMARDs are effective or as adjunctive therapy for disease that is refractory to conventional DMARD or biologic therapy.

▸ Combining a biologic agent with a conventional DMARD such as methotrexate is recommended for patients with moderate to high disease activity and for those who have had an inadequate response to a conventional DMARD alone.

▸ A targeted synthetic DMARD such as tofacitinib or baricitinib, with or without a conventional DMARD, can be used in patients with moderate or high disease activity.

Adverse Effects – In low doses, methotrexate is usually well tolerated, but it can cause stomatitis, anorexia, nausea, vomiting, abdominal cramps, fatigue, aminotransferase elevations, and hepatic fibrosis. Parenteral administration can decrease the GI adverse effects associated with oral formulations.

Methotrexate is an antifolate that is toxic to rapidly dividing cells; complete blood counts should be monitored during treatment.[1] Supplements containing folic acid or folinic acid are recommended to decrease adverse effects. Use of methotrexate has rarely been associated with localized lymphoma, which often regresses when the drug is stopped. Interstitial pneumonitis, which can be severe, occurs in <1% of patients. An increase in rheumatoid skin nodules and rare cases of cutaneous necrotizing vasculitis have been reported.

Pregnancy – Methotrexate is contraindicated for use during pregnancy. The drug should be stopped before conception for at least one and as many as three ovulatory cycles in women and for at least 3 months in men.

HYDROXYCHLOROQUINE — The antimalarial hydroxychloroquine is moderately effective for patients with low disease activity and is usually well tolerated. It is generally used in combination with other drugs, particularly methotrexate and sulfasalazine. In a randomized, double-blind, 48-week trial in 353 patients with active RA despite methotrexate therapy, adding hydroxychloroquine and sulfasalazine was noninferior to adding etanercept *(Enbrel)* in improving disease activity scores.[2]

Adverse Effects – Nausea and epigastric pain can occur, but serious adverse effects are rare. Hemolysis may occur in patients with glucose-6-phosphate dehydrogenase (G6PD) deficiency.

The most serious adverse effect of hydroxychloroquine is retinopathy. In the first 5 years of use, the risk is low if the daily dose is ≤5 mg/kg of actual body weight. A complete ophthalmologic exam is recommended before or soon after starting treatment to rule out underlying retinal disease, and annual screening should begin after 5 years of hydroxychloroquine use.[3,4]

Pregnancy – Use of hydroxychloroquine to treat rheumatoid arthritis should be avoided during pregnancy.

SULFASALAZINE — The aminosalicylate sulfasalazine has been shown to prevent joint erosions. Two to three months of therapy are often required for beneficial effects to become apparent. Sulfasalazine is frequently used in combination with hydroxychloroquine and/or methotrexate.

Adverse Effects – Nausea, anorexia, and rash are common. Use of the enteric-coated tablet formulation may decrease GI adverse effects. Serious reactions such as hepatitis, leukopenia, and agranulocytosis are rare and usually occur within the first 2-3 months of treatment. A lupus-like syndrome has been reported. Hemolysis may occur in patients with G6PD deficiency. Sperm counts may decrease during treatment, but return to normal after the drug is stopped.

Table 1. Some Conventional DMARDs for Rheumatoid Arthritis

Drug	Some Formulations
Methotrexate, oral – generic	2.5 mg tabs
Trexall (Duramed/Barr)	5, 7.5, 10, 15 mg tabs
Methotrexate, injectable – generic	25 mg/mL vials
Otrexup (Antares)	10, 12.5, 15, 17.5, 20, 22.5, 25 mg/0.4 mL auto-injectors
Rasuvo (Medac)	7.5 mg/0.15 mL, 10 mg/0.2 mL, 12.5 mg/0.25 mL, 15 mg/0.3 mL, 17.5 mg/0.35 mL, 20 mg/0.4 mL, 22.5 mg/0.45 mL, 25 mg/0.5 mL, 30 mg/0.6 mL auto-injectors
Hydroxychloroquine sulfate – generic	200 mg tabs
Plaquenil (Covis)	
Sulfasalazine – generic[7]	500 mg tabs
Azulfidine (Pfizer)[7]	
delayed-release – generic	500 mg enteric-coated delayed-release
Azulfidine EN-tabs (Pfizer)	tabs
Leflunomide – generic	10, 20 mg tabs
Arava (Sanofi)	10, 20 mg tabs

1. Dosage adjustment may be needed for hepatic or renal impairment.
2. Approximate WAC for 30 days' treatment with the lowest usual maintenance dosage. WAC = wholesaler acquisition cost or manufacturer's published price to wholesalers; WAC represents a published catalogue or list price and may not represent an actual transactional price. Source: AnalySource® Monthly. July 5, 2018. Reprinted with permission by First Databank, Inc. All rights reserved. ©2018. www.fdbhealth.com/policies/drug-pricing-policy.
3. In patients who cannot tolerate the single dose, methotrexate can be given in 3 divided doses. The dosage can be increased over 1-2 months up to 25 mg once/wk.
4. For initial treatment, an oral formulation of methotrexate should be used with *Otrexup*; an oral or SC formulation can be used with *Rasuvo*.

Pregnancy – Sulfasalazine is generally considered safe for use during pregnancy, but neural tube defects have been reported in infants born to women who took the drug during pregnancy. Sulfasalazine inhibits the absorption and metabolism of folic acid; pregnant women taking sulfasalazine may need higher doses of folic acid.

LEFLUNOMIDE — An oral inhibitor of pyrimidine synthesis, leflunomide (*Arava*, and generics) can decrease symptoms, limit joint damage, and improve motor function.[5]

Usual Adult Dosage[1]	Cost[2]
Initial: 7.5-10 mg PO once/wk[3]	$30.80
Maintenance: 7.5-25 mg PO once/wk[3]	83.00
Initial: 7.5 mg IM or SC once/wk[4,5]	5.80
Maintenance: 10-25 mg IM or SC once/wk[5,6]	649.80
	470.00
200-400 mg (max 5 mg/kg actual body weight) PO once/d	65.70
	155.70
Initial: 3-4 g/d in divided doses PO	22.30
Maintenance: 2 g/d in divided doses PO	181.10
	31.20
	236.50
Initial: 100 mg PO once/d x 3 d[8]	150.50
Maintenance: 10-20 mg PO once/d	1173.10

5. IM or SC methotrexate once weekly (in the same dose as the oral formulation) may be helpful for patients who have GI adverse effects from the oral formulation or lose benefit over time because of poor absorption. *Otrexup* and *Rasuvo* are only FDA-approved for subcutaneous use.
6. Maintenance dosage for *Rasuvo* is 7.5-30 mg SC once/week.
7. Not FDA-approved for treatment of rheumatoid arthritis.
8. Some expert clinicians omit initial therapy because of GI intolerability and risk of hepatotoxicity and myelosuppression.

Adverse Effects – Diarrhea occurs frequently with use of leflunomide. Reversible alopecia, weight loss, rash, myelosuppression, and aminotransferase elevations can also occur; monitoring of complete blood counts and liver enzymes is recommended. Anaphylaxis, Stevens-Johnson syndrome, interstitial lung disease, peripheral neuropathy, and leukocytoclastic vasculitis have occurred rarely.

Pregnancy – Leflunomide is carcinogenic and teratogenic in animals and is contraindicated for use during pregnancy. Leflunomide should be stopped before conception, and both men and women should take cholestyramine (*Questran*, and others) to bind and eliminate the drug. Without cholestyramine, it could take up to 2 years for serum concentrations of the drug to become undetectable.

AZATHIOPRINE — The immunosuppressive purine analog azathioprine (*Imuran*, and others) is sometimes used for patients with extra-articular disease such as rheumatoid vasculitis.

Adverse Effects – GI intolerance, hepatitis, and bone marrow suppression can occur. An increased risk of lymphoma has been reported.

Pregnancy – Adverse pregnancy outcomes have been reported in animal studies with azathioprine, but recent data in pregnant patients with inflammatory bowel disease suggest it is not associated with adverse birth outcomes.[6]

CYCLOSPORINE — Cyclosporine (*Neoral, Sandimmune,* and others) is an inhibitor of T-cell activation that has been shown to prevent joint erosions in RA. It is occasionally used as a second-line DMARD, but it interacts with many drugs.[7]

Adverse Effects – Hypertension and worsening renal function are common.

Pregnancy – No fetal adverse events were observed in animal studies. Premature births and low birth weight were observed in pregnant transplant patients given cyclosporine.

BIOLOGIC AGENTS AND JAK INHIBITORS

Biologic agents and Janus kinase (JAK) inhibitors are generally reserved for treatment of patients with moderate or high disease activity. Combining different biologic agents or a biologic agent and a JAK inhibitor increases the risk of infection and is not recommended.

TNF INHIBITORS — Tumor necrosis factor (TNF) is a pro-inflammatory cytokine present in the synovium of patients with RA. Five TNF inhibitors (adalimumab, certolizumab pegol, etanercept, golimumab, and infliximab) are FDA-approved for treatment of RA (see Table 2). All of them relieve RA symptoms and may be more effective than methotrexate alone in limiting joint destruction. TNF inhibitors have a faster onset of action than conventional DMARDs; some patients report substantial improvement after the first dose. Use of a TNF inhibitor in combination with methotrexate has synergistic beneficial effects.

Adverse Effects – Injection-site reactions are common with adalimumab, certolizumab pegol, etanercept, and golimumab. Infusion reactions can occur with infliximab and golimumab and can include fever, urticaria, dyspnea, and hypotension. Cytopenias can occur with all TNF inhibitors.

Patients treated with TNF inhibitors are at increased risk for serious infections, including reactivated and disseminated tuberculosis, invasive or disseminated fungal infection, and other opportunistic infections, such as those caused by *Legionella* and *Listeria*. Tuberculin skin testing or interferon-gamma release assay is recommended before starting and periodically during treatment. Inhibition of TNF has also been associated with reactivation of hepatitis B virus (HBV) in patients who are chronic carriers; serologic testing for active hepatitis B infection is recommended before starting treatment.[8]

Malignancies, especially lymphomas, have been reported with TNF inhibitors, but a cause-and-effect relationship has not been established. Patients with RA generally have an increased risk of lymphoma.

TNF inhibitors may rarely induce or exacerbate heart failure or induce a reversible lupus-like syndrome. Demyelinating conditions, including multiple sclerosis, optic neuritis, and Guillain-Barré syndrome, have occurred in patients being treated with these agents. Patients with pre-existing demyelinating conditions should not be treated with TNF inhibitors.

Table 2. Some Biologic Agents and JAK Inhibitors for Rheumatoid Arthritis

Drug	Some Formulations
Tumor Necrosis Factor (TNF) Inhibitors	
Adalimumab[3] – *Humira* (Abbvie)	10 mg/0.1 mL, 10 mg/0.2 mL, 20 mg/0.2 mL, 20 mg/0.4 mL syringes; 40 mg/0.8 mL prefilled pens and syringes
Certolizumab pegol – *Cimzia* (UCB)	200 mg single-dose vials; 200 mg/mL syringes
Etanercept – *Enbrel* (Amgen)	25 mg multiple-dose vials; 25 mg/0.5 mL, 50 mg/mL syringes; 50 mg/mL auto-injectors
Golimumab[4] – *Simponi* (Janssen)	50 mg/0.5 mL, 100 mg/mL syringes and auto-injectors
Simponi Aria	50 mg single-dose vials
Infliximab[4] – *Remicade* (Janssen) biosimilar[6] *Inflectra* (Celltrion) *Renflexis* (Merck)	100 mg single-dose vials
Interleukin (IL-6) Inhibitors	
Sarilumab[8] – *Kevzara* (Sanofi/Regeneron)	150 mg/1.14 mL, 200 mg/1.14 mL prefilled pens and syringes
Tocilizumab[8] – *Actemra* (Genentech)	80, 200, 400 mg single-dose vials
	162 mg/0.9 mL syringes

ER = extended-release
1. Dosage adjustment may be needed for hepatic or renal impairment.
2. Approximate WAC for 30 days' or 4 weeks' treatment with the usual dosage or lowest usual maintenance dosage (for a 70-kg patient treated with some parenteral drugs). WAC = wholesaler acquisition cost or manufacturer's published price to wholesalers; WAC represents a published catalogue or list price and may not represent an actual transactional price. Source: AnalySource® Monthly. July 5, 2018. Reprinted with permission by First Databank, Inc. All rights reserved. ©2018. www.fdbhealth.com/policies/drug-pricing-policy.
3. A biosimilar (adalimumab-adbm; *Cyltezo*) has been approved by the FDA but has not yet been marketed.

Usual Adult Dosage[1]	Cost[2]
40 mg SC q2 wks	$4872.00
Initial: 400 mg SC at 0, 2, and 4 wks Maintenance: 200 mg SC every other wk or 400 mg SC q4 wks	4044.30
25 mg SC 2x/wk or 50 mg SC once/wk	4872.00
50 mg SC once/month	4519.80
Initial: 2 mg/kg IV at 0 and 4 wks Maintenance: 2 mg/kg IV q8 wks	1733.60[5]
Initial: 3 mg/kg IV at 0, 2, and 6 wks Maintenance: 3 mg/kg IV q8 wks[7]	2784.70[5]
	1892.60[5]
	1506.80[5]
200 mg SC q2 wks	3159.00
Initial: 4 mg/kg IV q4 wks Maintenance: 8 mg/kg IV q4 wks	3276.10
Initial: 162 mg SC every other wk[9] Maintenance: 162 mg SC once/wk[10]	3938.90

4. FDA-approved only for use in combination with methotrexate.
5. Cost for 8 weeks' treatment.
6. Another biosimilar (infliximab-qbtx; *Ixifi*) has been approved by the FDA but has not yet been marketed.
7. Some patients may require higher doses (up to 10 mg/kg every 8 weeks) or more frequent doses (up to every 4 weeks).
8. FDA-approved for use in patients who have had an inadequate response or intolerance to ≥1 DMARDs.
9. Every week for patients weighing ≥100 kg.
10. In patients who weigh <100 kg, tocilizumab can be administered once every other week.

Continued on next page

Table 2. Some Biologic Agents and JAK Inhibitors for Rheumatoid Arthritis (continued)	
Drug	**Some Formulations**
Other Biologic Agents	
Rituximab[11] – *Rituxan* (Genentech)	100, 500 mg single-use vials
Abatacept – *Orencia* (BMS)	250 mg single-use vials 50 mg/0.4 mL, 87.5 mg/0.7 mL, 125 mg/mL syringes; 125 mg/mL auto-injectors
Anakinra[8] – *Kineret* (Sobi)	100 mg/0.67 mL syringes
Janus Kinase (JAK) Inhibitors	
Baricitinib[16] – *Olumiant* (Lilly)	2 mg tabs
Tofacitinib[17] – *Xeljanz* (Pfizer) *Xeljanz XR*	5 mg tabs 11 mg ER tabs

ER = extended-release
11. FDA-approved only for use with methotrexate in patients who have had an inadequate response to ≥1 TNF inhibitors.
12. Patients can be retreated every 4-6 months. IV methylprednisolone 100 mg or its equivalent infused 30 minutes before rituximab can reduce the incidence and severity of infusion reactions.
13. Cost of two 1000-mg doses.
14. Dose is 500 mg for patients weighing <60 kg, 750 mg for patients 60-100 kg, and 1000 mg for patients >100 kg.

Choice of a TNF Inhibitor – No head-to-head trials comparing TNF inhibitors are available, but they appear to be similar in efficacy. Patients who do not respond to one TNF inhibitor may respond to another. Etanercept has a rapid onset of action and a short half-life that makes toxicity, if it occurs, relatively short-lived. Infliximab and golimumab are FDA-approved only for use with methotrexate for treatment of RA. Golimumab has been shown to be effective in some patients who did not respond to infliximab or etanercept.[9]

IL-6 INHIBITORS — Sarilumab *(Kevzara)* is a human monoclonal antibody that inhibits the binding of interleukin-6 (IL-6) to its receptor. It has been effective in combination with methotrexate for treatment of patients whose disease had not responded to methotrexate or a TNF inhibitor. Given as monotherapy to patients who did not

Usual Adult Dosage[1]	Cost[2]
1000 mg IV twice, 2 wks apart[12]	$18,790.40[13]
500, 750, or 1000 mg IV at 0, 2, and 4 wks, then q4 wks[14]	2092.50
125 mg SC once/wk[15]	4131.00
100 mg SC once/d	4194.00
2 mg PO once/d	2054.70
5 mg PO bid	4296.30
11 mg PO once/d	4296.30

15. If administered after an initial IV loading dose, the first 125-mg SC injection should be given within a day of the IV loading dose (see footnote 12 for recommended loading dose).
16. FDA-approved for use in patients who have had an inadequate response to ≥1 TNF inhibitors.
17. FDA-approved for use in patients who have had an inadequate response or intolerance to methotrexate.

respond to or could not tolerate methotrexate, it was more effective than adalimumab.[10]

Infusion reactions, hypertension, neutropenia, elevated serum transaminase levels, and dyslipidemia can occur; monitoring of complete blood counts and liver enzymes is recommended. Serious infections and hypersensitivity reactions, including anaphylaxis, can occur.

Tocilizumab *(Actemra)* is a humanized monoclonal antibody that competitively inhibits the binding of the pro-inflammatory cytokine IL-6 to its receptor.[11] Clinical improvement has occurred in some RA patients as early as 2 weeks after starting therapy. In one clinical trial, tocilizumab monotherapy was significantly more effective than adalimumab monotherapy in reducing disease activity scores.[12] In patients with active RA despite methotrexate therapy, tocilizumab monotherapy may be as effective as combination therapy with methotrexate.[13] No studies comparing sarilumab with tocilizumab are available.

Adverse effects of tocilizumab are similar to those with sarilumab. An increase in lower GI tract perforations, especially in patients with a history of diverticulitis, has been reported with tocilizumab, but not with sarilumab to date.

OTHERS — Rituximab *(Rituxan)* is a genetically engineered chimeric murine/human monoclonal antibody that targets CD20, a B-cell-specific surface antigen. It has been effective in patients with RA who had an inadequate response to methotrexate and/or a TNF inhibitor.[14,15] Rituximab is only FDA-approved for use with methotrexate for treatment of RA.

Anaphylaxis and anaphylactoid reactions can occur within 2 hours of rituximab infusion; fatalities have been reported. Progressive multifocal leukoencephalopathy (PML) due to JC virus infection, which often causes death or severe neurological disability, and reactivation of HBV have been reported. Patients at high risk for hepatitis B infection should be screened for the disease before starting treatment. As with TNF inhibitors, antiviral prophylaxis against reactivation of HBV may be appropriate in some patients.[8]

Abatacept *(Orencia)* is a genetically engineered fusion protein that interferes with T-cell activation.[16] It can be used as monotherapy or in combination with a conventional DMARD. Given as monotherapy, it has been effective for treatment of RA that has not responded to methotrexate or TNF inhibitors.

Hypertension, headache, dizziness and, rarely, anaphylactoid reactions can occur within one hour after the start of an abatacept infusion. Abatacept may increase the risk of serious infections such as pneumonia, pyelonephritis, cellulitis, and diverticulitis.

Anakinra *(Kineret)* is a genetically engineered IL-1 receptor antagonist. It is the least commonly used biologic DMARD for RA because daily injections are required and there is limited evidence of its efficacy compared to other biologics.[1]

JAK INHIBITORS — **Tofacitinib** *(Xeljanz, Xeljanz XR)* is a synthetic oral inhibitor of Janus kinase (JAK), an important signaling mediator in various immune activation pathways.[17] In one clinical trial in 958 patients, first-line treatment with tofacitinib was superior to methotrexate in reducing signs and symptoms of RA and in slowing the progression of joint damage.[18] Added to methotrexate, its efficacy appears to be comparable to that of adalimumab plus methotrexate.[19]

Diarrhea, nasopharyngitis, upper respiratory tract infections, headache, and hypertension are common. Elevated hepatic transaminases, dyslipidemia, and cytopenias have been reported; periodic monitoring is recommended. Infections, especially herpes zoster and tuberculosis, can occur. An increased incidence of solid cancers was detected in short-term (≤12 months) clinical trials.

Baricitinib *(Olumiant)* is another synthetic oral JAK inhibitor. In clinical trials in patients with moderately to severely active RA that had not responded adequately to one or more TNF inhibitors, it was more effective than placebo.[20] No studies comparing baricitinib with tofacitinib are available.

Upper respiratory tract infections and nausea were the most common adverse effects reported in clinical trials. As with tofacitinib, serious infections such as tuberculosis and herpes zoster can occur. Thrombo-embolic events, malignancy, GI perforations, cytopenias, dyslipidemia, and elevated hepatic transaminases have also been reported.

PREGNANCY — No adequate data are available on the use of biologic agents and JAK inhibitors during pregnancy. TNF inhibitors are generally considered safe for use during pregnancy. Placental transfer of anti-TNF antibodies is higher in the late second and third trimesters, especially with infliximab, adalimumab, and golimumab. None of these drugs are contraindicated for use during pregnancy.[21]

COMBINATION THERAPY

Combination treatment is particularly useful for patients with a long duration of disease or clinical features that indicate a poor prognosis, such as a positive rheumatoid factor or anti-CCP test, functional limitations, extra-articular disease, or bony erosions.

A combination of 2 or 3 conventional DMARDs or a conventional DMARD and a biologic agent or JAK inhibitor may be more effective than monotherapy without causing a significant increase in toxicity. The combination of methotrexate and a biologic agent has been typically more effective than methotrexate alone in achieving and maintaining minimal disease activity. Combining different biologic agents or a biologic agent and a JAK inhibitor increases the risk of infection and is not recommended. Use of leflunomide with methotrexate increases the risk of hepatotoxicity.

CORTICOSTEROIDS

Oral corticosteroids can relieve joint symptoms and control systemic manifestations. A short course of a low-dose corticosteroid is commonly used for symptomatic relief until the beneficial effects of DMARDs become apparent. In patients with early RA, prednisone 7.5 mg daily has been reported to reduce radiographic progression, and the addition of daily prednisone 10 mg to methotrexate has been shown to reduce erosive joint damage and increase the likelihood of remission compared to methotrexate alone,[22] but most clinicians do not use long-term corticosteroids because of their many adverse effects. High doses of corticosteroids may be needed to control severe systemic manifestations of RA, such as pericarditis or vasculitis, but with the use of methotrexate and biologic agents, these conditions are now uncommon.

Intra-articular injection of a corticosteroid such as triamcinolone (*Aristospan*, and others) or methylprednisolone *(Depomedrol)* can often relieve an acutely inflamed rheumatoid joint with minimal adverse effects; injecting one or two joints in a patient with limited disease is probably underutilized.

NSAIDS

Nonsteroidal anti-inflammatory drugs (NSAIDs), including COX 2-selective celecoxib (*Celebrex*, and generics), have immediate analgesic and anti-inflammatory effects. Since conventional DMARDs and biologic agents have been found to be effective and safe for long-term use, NSAIDs are now used mainly as bridge drugs for symptom relief. No oral NSAID is consistently more effective than any other for treatment of RA, but some patients who do not respond to or tolerate one may respond to or tolerate another.[23] Topical diclofenac *(Voltaren Gel, Pennsaid)* is FDA-approved only for use in osteoarthritis, but it may be helpful in some patients with RA who have isolated symptomatic joints.[24]

1. JA Singh et al. 2015 American College of Rheumatology guideline for the treatment of rheumatoid arthritis. Arthritis Rheumatol 2016; 68:1.
2. JR O'Dell et al. Therapies for active rheumatoid arthritis after methotrexate failure. N Engl J Med 2013; 369:307.
3. MF Marmor et al. Recommendations on screening for chloroquine and hydroxychloroquine retinopathy. Ophthalmology 2016; 123:1386.
4. N Abdulaziz et al. Hydroxychloroquine: balancing the need to maintain therapeutic levels with ocular safety: an update. Curr Opin Rheumatol 2018; 30:249.
5. N Alcorn et al. Benefit-risk assessment of leflunomide: an appraisal of leflunomide in rheumatoid arthritis 10 years after licensing. Drug Saf 2009; 32:1123.
6. Drugs for inflammatory bowel disease. Med Lett Drugs Ther 2018; 60:107.
7. Drug interactions from The Medical Letter. Available at: www.secure.medicalletter.org/subDIO. Accessed July 19, 2018.
8. KR Reddy et al. American Gastroenterological Association Institute guideline on the prevention and treatment of hepatitis B virus reactivation during immunosuppressive drug therapy. Gastroenterology 2015; 148:215.
9. JS Smolen et al. Insights into the efficacy of golimumab plus methotrexate in patients with active rheumatoid arthritis who discontinued prior anti-tumour necrosis factor therapy: post-hoc analyses from the GO-AFTER study. Ann Rheum Dis 2014; 73:1811.
10. Sarilumab (Kevzara) for rheumatoid arthritis. Med Lett Drugs Ther 2017; 59:134.

11. Tocilizumab (Actemra) for rheumatoid arthritis. Med Lett Drugs Ther 2010; 52:47.
12. C Gabay et al. Tocilizumab monotherapy versus adalimumab monotherapy for treatment of rheumatoid arthritis (ADACTA): a randomised, double-blind, controlled phase 4 trial. Lancet 2013; 381:1541.
13. M Dougados et al. Adding tocilizumab or switching to tocilizumab monotherapy in methotrexate inadequate responders: 24-week symptomatic and structural results of a 2-year randomised controlled strategy trial in rheumatoid arthritis (ACT-RAY). Ann Rheum Dis 2013; 72:43.
14. Rituximab (Rituxan) for rheumatoid arthritis. Med Lett Drugs Ther 2006; 48:34.
15. SB Cohen et al. Rituximab for rheumatoid arthritis refractory to anti-tumor necrosis factor therapy: results of a multicenter, randomized, double-blind, placebo-controlled, phase III trial evaluating primary efficacy and safety at twenty-four weeks. Arthritis Rheum 2006; 54:2793.
16. Abatacept (Orencia) for rheumatoid arthritis. Med Lett Drugs Ther 2006; 48:17.
17. Tofacitinib (Xeljanz) for rheumatoid arthritis. Med Lett Drugs Ther 2013; 55:1.
18. EB Lee et al. Tofacitinib versus methotrexate in rheumatoid arthritis. N Engl J Med 2014; 370:2377.
19. RF van Vollenhoven et al. Tofacitinib or adalimumab versus placebo in rheumatoid arthritis. N Engl J Med 2012; 367:508.
20. Baricitinib (Olumiant) for rheumatoid arthritis. Med Lett Drugs Ther 2018; 60:120.
21. ML Krause and A Makol. Management of rheumatoid arthritis during pregnancy: challenges and solutions. Open Access Rheumatol 2016; 8:23.
22. MF Bakker et al. Low-dose prednisone inclusion in a methotrexate-based, tight control strategy for early rheumatoid arthritis: a randomized trial. Ann Intern Med 2012; 156:329.
23. Nonopioid drugs for pain. Med Lett Drugs Ther 2018; 60:24.
24. Diclofenac gel for osteoarthritis. Med Lett Drugs Ther 2008; 50:31.

CHOICE OF
Contraceptives

Original publication date – October 2018

Intrauterine devices (IUDs) and the etonogestrel implant are the most effective reversible contraceptive methods available. Hormonal oral contraceptives, patches, rings, and injectables are also highly effective in preventing pregnancy. When used alone, barrier and fertility-based methods generally have higher failure rates than other methods.[1-3]

COMBINATION ORAL CONTRACEPTIVES — Most oral contraceptives available in the US consist of a combination of the estrogen ethinyl estradiol and a progestin. The amount of estrogen and progestin in these pills has been reduced over the years to decrease the incidence of adverse effects. Formulations that contain ≤20 mcg of ethinyl estradiol are effective, but they can cause irregular, frequent, or prolonged bleeding.[4]

Monophasic oral contraceptives contain fixed doses of estrogen and progestin in each active pill. **Multiphasic** oral contraceptives vary the dose of one or both hormones throughout the 28-day cycle. Many multiphasic pills deliver a lower total hormone dose per cycle than monophasic pills, but there is no convincing evidence that they cause fewer adverse effects.

Most traditional oral contraceptives contain 21 active tablets and 7 placebo (or iron) tablets, resulting in 13 scheduled withdrawal bleeds per year. Regimens with **fewer hormone-free days** (2-4 placebo or iron tablets per 28-day cycle) or **continuous** or **extended cycles** with fewer

---

Recommendations

Contraception

► Intrauterine devices (IUDs) and the etonogestrel implant are highly effective in preventing pregnancy and require no adherence. They are generally the most cost-effective of all reversible contraceptives.

► Oral contraceptives containing estrogen (≤35 mcg of ethinyl estradiol) and a progestin are also highly effective and have noncontraceptive benefits such as a reduced risk of endometrial and epithelial ovarian cancer.

► Barrier contraceptives (condoms, diaphragms, cervical caps, spermicides, sponges) generally have higher failure rates than IUDs and hormonal contraceptives, but they have fewer systemic adverse effects.

► Failure rates with fertility awareness-based methods are high.

Emergency Contraception

► The copper-containing IUD *(ParaGard)* is the most effective method of emergency contraception.

► Oral ulipristal acetate *(Ella)*, available only by prescription, is the most effective hormonal option for emergency contraception.

► Single-dose levonorgestrel is available over the counter with no age restriction for emergency contraception.

---

withdrawal bleeds per year are commonly used now. Extended-cycle contraceptives may be beneficial for women who have dysmenorrhea, premenstrual syndrome, or premenstrual dysphoric disorder (PMDD).[5]

Noncontraceptive Benefits – Women who take combination oral contraceptives have a reduced risk of endometrial and epithelial ovarian cancer.[6] This benefit is detectable within the first year of use and appears to persist for years after discontinuation. Other benefits include a reduction in bleeding and dysmenorrhea, a lower incidence of ectopic pregnancy and benign breast disease, and an increase in hemoglobin concentrations.[7] Many women also benefit from the convenience of menstrual regularity. Combination oral contraceptives increase sex hormone binding globulin and decrease free testosterone concentrations, which may lead to improvements in hirsutism and acne.[8] Some combination oral contraceptives are FDA-approved for treatment of acne or PMDD. Combination oral contraceptives are also often used off-label to treat polycystic ovary syndrome and endometriosis pain.

Choice of a Progestin – Desogestrel, norgestimate, and drospirenone have less androgenic activity and are claimed to improve acne more than older progestins. Combination oral contraceptives containing drospirenone, a synthetic progestin with antiandrogenic and antimineralocorticoid activity, have been shown to improve PMDD symptoms, hirsutism, and acne. Their efficacy appears to be similar to that of other combination oral contraceptives for treatment of acne; how they compare to other combination oral contraceptives for treatment of PMDD and hirsutism is unclear.[9,10]

Adverse Effects – Combination oral contraceptives can cause headache, nausea, bloating, and breast tenderness and enlargement. Breakthrough bleeding or spotting is common with low-dose ($\leq$20 mcg) ethinyl estradiol formulations and extended-cycle or continuous regimens, particularly during the initial cycles. Drospirenone can cause hyperkalemia.

Formulations of combination oral contraceptives containing $\geq$50 mcg of ethinyl estradiol have been associated with increased risks of myocardial infarction and ischemic stroke, particularly in women who smoked or had uncontrolled hypertension; these risks are reduced with formulations that contain $\leq$35 mcg of ethinyl estradiol.

The risk of venous thromboembolism (VTE) is 2-3 times higher in women taking combination oral contraceptives that contain $\leq$35 mcg of ethinyl estradiol than in nonusers; this risk is lower, however, than the risk of VTE associated with pregnancy. The risk of VTE is higher in women who are $\geq$40 years old or obese, and in those who smoke, have an inherited thrombophilia, or a history of VTE. Some progestins (desogestrel and drospirenone) have been associated with a higher risk of VTE compared to levonorgestrel.[11,12]

Table 1. Efficacy of Contraceptives for Pregnancy Prevention

Method	Failure Rate[1]	
	Typical Use	Perfect Use
Permanent Contraception		
Tubal occlusion	0.5%	0.5%
Vasectomy	0.15%	0.10%
Implant (etonogestrel)		
Nexplanon (Merck)	0.1%	0.1%
Intrauterine devices (IUDs)		
Copper-containing IUD		
ParaGard (Cooper Surgical)	0.8%	0.6%
Levonorgestrel-releasing IUDs		
Kyleena (Bayer)	0.2%	0.2%
Liletta (Allergan/Medicines 360)	0.1%	0.1%
Mirena (Bayer)	0.1%	0.1%
Skyla (Bayer)	0.4%	0.3%
Injectable (medroxyprogesterone acetate)		
Depo-Provera (Pfizer)	6%	0.2%
Combination oral contraceptives	7%[2]	0.3%[2]

OTC = over the counter; PID = pelvic inflammatory disease; STIs = sexually transmitted infections
1. Estimated percentage who experience an unintended pregnancy during first year of use; adapted from J Trussell and ARA Aiken. Contraceptive efficacy. In RA Hatcher et al, Contraceptive Technology: Twenty-first revised edition, New York, NY: Ayer Company Publishers 2018.

Some Advantages	Some Adverse Effects/Disadvantages
Long-term contraception; no patient compliance required	Potential for surgical complications; regret among young women; reversal often not possible
Long-term contraception; no patient compliance required	Pain at surgical site; regret among young men; reversal often not possible
Convenience; long-term contraception; no patient compliance required; rapid return of fertility after removal	Irregular bleeding; removal complications; requires in-office insertion procedure
Convenience; long-term contraception; no patient compliance required; rapid return of fertility after removal	Rare uterine perforation; risk of infection with insertion; anemia; requires in-office insertion procedure; available only by prescription
Effective for 10 years; nonhormonal	Irregular/heavy bleeding and dysmenorrhea
Decreased menstrual bleeding and dysmenorrhea; amenorrhea after 1 year in 6% with *Skyla*, 12% with *Kyleena*, 19% with *Liletta*, and 20% with *Mirena*; smaller T-frame and narrower insertion tube with *Kyleena* and *Skyla*	Irregular bleeding in first 3-6 months; headache; nausea; acne; ovarian cysts
Convenience; same benefits as progestin-only oral contraceptives	Delayed return to fertility; irregular bleeding and amenorrhea; weight gain; may decrease bone mineral density; available only by prescription
Decreased risk of ovarian and endometrial cancer, PID, and dysmenorrhea	Increased risk of thromboembolism; nausea; headache; available only by prescription

2. Based on combined data with combination and progestin-only contraceptives. Failure rates with progestin-only oral contraceptives may be higher.

Continued on next page

Table 1. Efficacy of Contraceptives for Pregnancy Prevention (continued)

Method	Failure Rate[1]	
	Typical Use	Perfect Use
Progestin-only oral contraceptives	7%[2]	0.3%[2]
Transdermal		
Xulane (Mylan)	7%	0.3%
Vaginal rings		
Annovera (Population Council)	See footnote 3	
NuvaRing (Merck)	7%	0.3%
Diaphragm with spermicide	17%	16%
Cervical cap	16-32%[4]	9-26%[4]
FemCap (FemCap)		
Condom without spermicide		
Female	21%	5%
Male	13%	2%

OTC = over the counter; PID = pelvic inflammatory disease; STIs = sexually transmitted infections
3. In clinical trials, summarized in the package insert, the pregnancy rate was 2.98 per 100 woman-years of *Annovera* use. *Annovera* is expected to be available in late 2019.

Some Advantages	Some Adverse Effects/Disadvantages
Decreased risk of PID, iron-deficiency anemia, and dysmenorrhea; safe in those with cardiovascular risk	Irregular, unpredictable bleeding; may worsen acne; must be taken at same time every day; available only by prescription
Convenience of once-weekly application; same benefits as combination oral contraceptives	Increased estrogen exposure compared to oral contraceptives; dysmenorrhea and breast discomfort may be more frequent than with combination oral contraceptives; application site reactions; detachment; available only by prescription
Convenience of once-monthly insertion; excellent cycle control; rapid return to fertility after removal	Discomfort; vaginal discharge; available only by prescription
May reduce risk of cervical cancer	High failure rate; cervical irritation; increased risk of urinary tract infection and toxic shock syndrome; some require fitting by healthcare professional; may be difficult to obtain; available only by prescription
Effective for 48 hours; reapplication of spermicide not required; can be used for up to 2 years	High failure rate; cervical irritation; pap smear abnormalities; limited sizes available; increased risk of toxic shock syndrome; may be difficult to obtain; available only by prescription
Protection against STIs; covers external genitalia; available OTC	High failure rate; difficult to insert; poor acceptability
Protection against STIs; available OTC	High failure rate; allergic reactions; poor acceptability; breakage possible

4. J Trussell and KA Guthrie. Choosing a contraceptive: efficacy, safety, and personal consideration. In: RA Hatcher et al. Contraceptive Technology: 20th revised edition. New York, NY: Ardent Media 2011.

Continued on next page

Table 1. Efficacy of Contraceptives for Pregnancy Prevention (continued)		
	Failure Rate[1]	
Method	**Typical Use**	**Perfect Use**
Sponge	14%/27%[5]	9%/20%[5]
Today (Mayer)		
Withdrawal	20%	4%
Spermicide alone	21%	16%
Fertility awareness-based methods	15%	–
Ovulation method	23%	3%
TwoDay method	14%	4%
Standard Days method	12%	5%
Natural Cycles mobile app	6.8%[6]	1.8%[6]
Symptothermal method	2%	0.4%
No method	85%	85%

OTC = over the counter; PID = pelvic inflammatory disease; STIs = sexually transmitted infections
5. In nulliparous/parous women.

Data linking the use of combination oral contraceptives and an increased risk of breast cancer are conflicting. A recent study found a small increase in the risk of breast cancer among current and long-term users.[13]

Data on the effects of combination oral contraceptives on mood are conflicting. A recent study found that use of hormonal contraceptives was associated with a small increase in subsequent first antidepressant use compared to nonusers; the risk was higher in adolescents than in older women.[14]

Contraindications – Estrogen-containing contraceptives are contraindicated for use in women who are pregnant or have a history of breast cancer, liver disease (tumor, acute viral hepatitis, or severe cirrhosis), or undiagnosed abnormal uterine bleeding. They are also contraindicated for use in women who are at high risk of thrombotic disease, including those who are ≥35 years old and smoke, have diabetes or migraine

Some Advantages	Some Adverse Effects/Disadvantages
No fitting required; provides 24 hours of protection; available OTC	High failure rate; contraindicated during menses; increased risk of toxic shock syndrome; less effective in nulliparous women
No drugs or devices	High failure rate
Available OTC	High failure rate; local irritation; must be reapplied with repeat intercourse
No drugs or devices	High failure rate; may be difficult to learn; requires periods of abstinence or use of a barrier contraceptive method
—	—

6. RG Simmons et al. JMIR Res Protoc 2017; 6:e5.

headache, and those with VTE, coronary artery or cerebrovascular disease, thrombogenic valvular or rhythm diseases, hypercoagulopathies, uncontrolled hypertension, or headaches with focal neurological symptoms.[3,15] Progestin-only or nonhormonal methods are preferred in women at increased risk of cardiovascular or thromboembolic events. Combination oral contraceptives should not be started <21 days postpartum.

Drug Interactions – Drugs that induce hepatic enzyme activity, such as rifampin, antiretrovirals, anticonvulsants, and St. John's wort, can increase the metabolism of hormonal contraceptives and decrease their effectiveness. Recent studies suggest that concurrent use of non-rifamycin antibiotics does not reduce the efficacy of hormonal contraceptives.[16]

PROGESTIN-ONLY ORAL CONTRACEPTIVES — All progestin-only pills (also called minipills) available in the US contain norethindrone. They are taken daily without a hormone-free interval and are used predominantly by breastfeeding women and those in whom estrogen is poorly tolerated or contraindicated. They should ideally be started on the first day of menses; backup contraception is recommended for women who start treatment >5 days after menses onset. Progestin-only pills commonly cause irregular bleeding and they may worsen acne. Taking the pill at the same time each day is crucial for prevention of pregnancy and breakthrough bleeding.

TRANSDERMAL PATCH — *Xulane*, a generic version of the *Ortho Evra* patch (no longer marketed), delivers an average daily dose of 35 mcg of ethinyl estradiol and 0.15 mg of norelgestromin. A new patch is applied to the buttock, lower abdomen, back, or upper outer arm each week for 3 weeks, followed by one patch-free week. Its efficacy is similar to that of combination oral contraceptives, although it may be less effective in women who weigh ≥90 kg. The adverse effects and risks of the patch are similar to those of combination oral contraceptives, but patch users are exposed to higher average levels of estrogen than users of combination oral contraceptives containing 30-35 mcg of ethinyl estradiol. Compliance may be improved compared to oral contraceptives, but breakthrough bleeding is more common during the first 2 cycles. Skin irritation at the application site can occur and may lead to discontinuation.

VAGINAL RINGS — *NuvaRing* delivers a daily dose of 15 mcg of ethinyl estradiol and 0.12 mg of etonogestrel, the active metabolite of desogestrel. It is placed intravaginally by the patient and left in place for 3 weeks, followed by one ring-free week. The ring can be left in place for a maximum of 4 weeks, reducing or eliminating the number of ring-free days. A new ring is used for every 4-week cycle. If the ring is removed for more than 3 hours, backup contraception should be used until the ring has been in place for 7 consecutive days. Its efficacy is similar to that of combination oral contraceptives, but users report less nausea, acne, irritability, and depression.

Another vaginal ring *(Annovera)* has recently been approved by the FDA; it is expected to be available in late 2019. The ring delivers an average daily dose of 13 mcg of ethinyl estradiol and 0.15 mg of segesterone acetate. It is placed intravaginally by the patient and left in place for 3 weeks, followed by one ring-free week. Unlike *NuvaRing*, the same *Annovera* ring can be reinserted every 4 weeks for up to one year. The efficacy of *Annovera* in women with a BMI >29 kg/m^2 has not been established. No head-to-head trials comparing *Annovera* with *NuvaRing* are available.

Both rings offer excellent cycle control and a rapid return to fertility after removal. Reasons for discontinuation have included headaches, vaginal discharge, and device-related discomfort.

INJECTABLE CONTRACEPTIVE — The injectable progestin medroxyprogesterone acetate (MPA) is effective and eliminates the need for daily adherence. MPA is injected IM (*Depo-Provera*, and generics) or SC *(Depo-SubQ Provera 104)* once every 3 months. Amenorrhea is common and irregular bleeding can occur. Weight gain, headache, and decreases in bone mineral density (BMD) have been reported. Because of the risk of bone loss, the labeling for each MPA product recommends stopping it after 2 years of use unless no acceptable alternative is available, but the American College of Obstetricians and Gynecologists has urged practitioners to continue the injections after 2 years when they judge such use to be appropriate. Decreases in BMD appear to be reversible after stopping the drug in most women.[17] The return of fertility can be delayed for 6-12 months (median 10 months) after the last injection.

SUBDERMAL IMPLANT — *Nexplanon*, a single-rod implant containing the progestin etonogestrel, is placed under the skin on the inside of the non-dominant upper arm.[18] It releases 60-70 mcg/day of etonogestrel initially, 30-40 mcg/day at the end of the second year, and 25-30 mcg/day at the end of the third year. Implants, once placed, provide long-term protection against pregnancy and require no adherence other than an office visit for replacement after 4 years. Fertility returns

Table 2. Some Oral Hormonal Contraceptives[1,2]

Monophasic Combinations

Ethynodiol diacetate/ethinyl estradiol (1 mg/50 mcg)
Kelnor 1/50 (Teva)[3]

Norgestrel[4]/ethinyl estradiol (0.5 mg/50 mcg)
Ogestrel 0.5/50 (Teva)[3]

Ethynodiol diacetate/ethinyl estradiol (1 mg/35 mcg)
Kelnor 1/35 (Teva)[3]
Pirmella 1/35 (Lupin)[3]
Zovia 1/35E (Mayne)[3]

Norethindrone/ethinyl estradiol (1 mg/35 mcg)
Alyacen 1/35 (Glenmark)[3]
Cyclafem 1/35 (Par)[3]
Dasetta 1/35 (NorthStar)[3]
Nortrel 1/35 (Teva)[3,5]
Ortho-Novum 1/35 (Janssen)[3]

Norethindrone/ethinyl estradiol (0.5 mg/35 mcg)
Brevicon (Allergan)[3]
Necon 0.5/35 (Mayne)[3]
Nortrel (Teva)[3,5]
Wera (NorthStar)[3]

Norethindrone/ethinyl estradiol (0.4 mg/35 mcg)
Balziva (Teva)[3]
Briellyn (Glenmark)[3]
Philith (NorthStar)[3]
Vyfemla (Lupin)[3]

Norgestimate/ethinyl estradiol (0.25 mg/35 mcg)
Femyor (Amneal)[3]
Mili (Aurobindo)[3]
Mono-Linyah (NorthStar)[3]
MonoNessa (Teva)[3]
Ortho-Cyclen (Janssen)[3]
Previfem (Par)[3]

Fe = contains iron
1. Different progestins are not equivalent on a milligram-to-milligram basis.
2. Oral contraceptives can cost $15-50/month without commercial or government insurance. Many are available at no charge or at a lower cost with commercial or government insurance.
3. Packaged as active tablets for 21 days and placebo for 7 days.
4. The progestin norgestrel contains two isomers; only levonorgestrel is bioactive. The amount of norgestrel in each tablet is twice the amount of levonorgestrel.
5. Packaged as active tablets for 21 days.

Continued on next page

Table 2. Some Oral Hormonal Contraceptives[1,2] (continued)

Monophasic Combinations (continued)

Norgestimate/ethinyl estradiol (0.25 mg/35 mcg) (continued)
Sprintec (Teva)[3]
VyLibra (Afaxys)[3]

Desogestrel/ethinyl estradiol (0.15 mg/30 mcg)
Apri (Teva)[3]
Cyreq Eq (Afaxys)[3]
Emoquette (Par)[3]
Enskyce (Lupin)[3]
Juleber (NorthStar)[3]
Reclipsen (Teva)[3]

Drospirenone/ethinyl estradiol (3 mg/30 mcg)
Ocella (Teva)[3]
Safyral (Bayer)[6,7]
Tydemy (Lupin)[6,7]
Yasmin (Bayer)[3]
Zarah (Mayne)[3]

Levonorgestrel/ethinyl estradiol (0.15 mg/30 mcg)
Chateal Eq (Afaxys)[3]
Kurvelo (Lupin)[3]
Levora 0.15/30 (Mayne)[3]
Lillow (Amneal)[3]
Marlissa (Glenmark)[3]
Portia (Teva)[3]

Norethindrone acetate/ethinyl estradiol (1.5 mg/30 mcg)
Blisovi Fe 1.5/30 (Lupin)[9]
Larin Fe 1.5/30 (NorthStar)[8,9]
Loestrin Fe 1.5/30 (Teva)[8,9]
Microgestin Fe 1.5/30 (Mayne)[8,9]
Junel Fe 1.5/30 (Teva)[8,9]

Norgestrel[4]/ethinyl estradiol (0.3 mg/30 mcg)
Cryselle (Teva)[3]
Elinest (NorthStar)[3]

Fe = contains iron
6. Also contains 451 mcg of levomefolate calcium per tablet. Addition of levomefolate increases folate levels in order to reduce the risk of a neural tube defect in a fetus conceived during or shortly after oral contraceptive use.
7. Packaged as active tablets for 21 days and levomefolate calcium alone for 7 days.
8. Also available in a 21-day regimen that does not contain iron.
9. Packaged as active tablets for 21 days and ferrous fumarate tablets for 7 days.

Continued on next page

Table 2. Some Oral Hormonal Contraceptives[1,2] (continued)

Monophasic Combinations (continued)

Norgestrel[4]/ethinyl estradiol (0.3 mg/30 mcg) (continued)
Low-Ogestrel (Mayne)[3]

Drospirenone/ethinyl estradiol (3 mg/20 mcg)
Beyaz (Bayer)[6,10-12]
Gianvi (Teva)[13]
Loryna (Xiromed)[11,13]
Nikki (Lupin)[11,13]
Yaz (Bayer)[11-13]

Levonorgestrel/ethinyl estradiol (0.9 mg/20 mcg)
Amethyst (Teva)[12]

Levonorgestrel/ethinyl estradiol (0.1 mg/20 mcg)
Aviane (Teva)[3]
Balcoltra (Avion)[3]
Falmina (NorthStar)[3]
Larissia (Amneal)[3]
Lessina (Teva)[3]
Lutera (Mayne)[3]
Orsythia (Par)[3]
Sronyx (Mayne)[3]

Norethindrone acetate/ethinyl estradiol (1 mg/20 mcg)
Blisovi Fe 1/20 (Lupin)[9,14]
Junel Fe 1/20 (Teva)[8,9,14]
Larin Fe 1/20 (NorthStar)[8,9,14]
Loestrin Fe 1/20 (Teva)[8,9]
Melodetta 24 Fe (Amneal)[14,15]
Mibelas 24 Fe (Lupin)[14,15]
Microgestin Fe 1/20 (Mayne)[8,9]
Minastrin Fe 1/20 (Allergan)[14,15]
Taytulla (Allergan)[14,16]

Fe = contains iron
10. Packaged as active tablets for 24 days and levomefolate calcium alone for 4 days.
11. Also FDA-approved for moderate acne.
12. Also FDA-approved for treatment of premenstrual dysphoric disorder (PMDD).
13. Packaged as active tablets for 24 days and placebo for 4 days.
14. Available in a 28-day regimen, with active pills for 24 days and ferrous fumarate for 4 days.
15. Chewable tablets.
16. Capsules.

Continued on next page

Table 2. Some Oral Hormonal Contraceptives[1,2] (continued)

Multiphasic Combinations

Norethindrone/ethinyl estradiol (0.5/35, 0.75/35, 1/35 mg/mcg)
   Alyacen 7/7/7 (Glenmark)[3]
   Cyclafem 7/7/7 (Par)[3]
   Dasetta 7/7/7 (NorthStar)[3]
   Nortrel 7/7/7 (Teva)[3]
   Ortho-Novum 7/7/7 (Janssen)[3]
   Pirmella 7/7/7 (Lupin)[3]

Norethindrone/ethinyl estradiol (0.5/35, 1/35, 0.5/35 mg/mcg)
   Aranelle 7/9/5 (Teva)[3]
   Leena 7/9/5 (Mayne)[3]

Norgestimate/ethinyl estradiol (0.18/35, 0.215/35, 0.25/35 mg/mcg)
   Ortho Tri-Cyclen (Janssen)[3,11]
   Tri Femynor (Amneal)[3,11]
   Tri-Linyah (NorthStar)[3,11]
   Tri-Mili (Aurobindo)[3,11]
   Tri-Previfem (Par)[3,11]
   Tri-Sprintec (Teva)[3,11]
   TriNessa 28 (Teva)[3,11]

Desogestrel/ethinyl estradiol (0.1/25, 0.125/25, 0.15/25 mg/mcg)
   Caziant (Mayne)[3]
   Cyclessa (Merck)[3]
   Velivet (Teva)[3]

Norgestimate/ethinyl estradiol (0.18/25, 0.215/25, 0.25/25 mg/mcg)
   Ortho Tri-Cyclen Lo (Janssen)[3]
   Tri-Lo-Marzia (Lupin)[3]
   Tri-Lo-Sprintec (Teva)[3]
   TriNessa Lo (Teva)[3]

Norethindrone acetate/ethinyl estradiol (1/20, 1/30, 1/35 mg/mcg)
   Estrostep Fe (Allergan)[9,11]
   Tilia Fe (Mayne)[9,11]
   Tri-Legest Fe (Teva)[8,9,11]

Desogestrel/ethinyl estradiol (0.15/20, 0/0, 0/10 mg/mcg)
   Azurette (Mayne)[17]

Fe = contains iron
17. Packaged as active tablets for 26 days (24 days of the combination and 2 days of ethinyl estradiol
    only) and placebo (or ferrous fumarate for *Lo Loestrin Fe*) for 2 days.

Continued on next page

Table 2. Some Oral Hormonal Contraceptives[1,2] (continued)

Multiphasic Combinations (continued)

Desogestrel/ethinyl estradiol (0.15/20, 0/0, 0/10 mg/mcg) (continued)
Bekyree (Lupin)[17]
Kariva (Teva)[17]
Mircette (Teva)[17]
Pimtrea (NorthStar)[17]
Viorele (Glenmark)[17]

Levonorgestrel/ethinyl estradiol (0.05/30, 0.075/40, 0.125/30 mg/mcg)
Enpresse (Teva)[3]
Levonest (NorthStar)[3]
Myzilra (Par)[3]
Trivora (Mayne)[3]

Norethindrone acetate/ethinyl estradiol (1/10, 0/10 mg/mcg)
Lo Loestrin Fe (Allergan)[17]

Dienogest/estradiol valerate (0/3, 2/2, 3/2, 0/1 mg/mg)
Natazia (Bayer)[18]

Extended-Cycle

Levonorgestrel/ethinyl estradiol (0.15 mg/30 mcg)
Jolessa (Teva)[19]
Setlakin (NorthStar)[19]
Quasense (Teva)[19]

Levonorgestrel/ethinyl estradiol (0.15/30, 0/10 mg/mcg)
Amethia (Mayne)[20]
Ashlyna (Glenmark)[20]
Camrese (Teva)[20]
Daysee (Lupin)[20]
Seasonique (Teva)[20]

Levonorgestrel/ethinyl estradiol (0.1/20, 0/10 mg/mcg)
Amethia Lo (Mayne)[20]
Camrese Lo (Teva)[20]
LoSeasonique (Teva)[20]

Levonorgestrel/ethinyl estradiol (0.15/20, 0.15/25, 0.15/30, 0/10 mg/mcg)
Fayosim (Lupin)[20]
Rivelsa (Teva)[20]
Quartette (Teva)[20]

Fe = contains iron
18. Packaged as active tablets for 26 days and placebo for 2 days. Also FDA-approved for treatment of heavy menstrual bleeding in women without organic pathology.
19. Packaged as a 91-day regimen: active tablets for 84 days and placebo for 7 days.
20. Packaged as a 91-day regimen: 84 days of the combination and 7 days of ethinyl estradiol only.

Continued on next page

Table 2. Some Oral Hormonal Contraceptives[1,2] (continued)
Progestin-Only
Norethindrone (0.35 mg)
Camila (Mayne)[21]
Deblitane (NorthStar)[21]
Errin (Mayne)[21]
Heather (Glenmark)[21]
Incassia (Aurobindo)[21]
Jencycla (Lupin)[21]
Jolivette (Teva)[21]
Nora-BE (Teva)[21]
Norlyda (Amneal)[21]
Ortho Micronor (Janssen)[21]
Sharobel (NorthStar)[21]

Fe = contains iron
21. Packaged as active tablets for 28 days.

rapidly after removal.[19] As with other progestin-based methods, bleeding irregularities are common.

INTRAUTERINE DEVICES (IUDs) — The 5 IUDs available in the US are all highly effective in preventing pregnancy. Once inserted, they require no adherence (other than an office visit for replacement) and provide convenient, long-term contraception; fertility is restored upon removal. IUDs are considered safe for use in most women, including adolescents and nulliparous women.[20,21] All of the levonorgestrel-releasing IUDs can reduce dysmenorrhea. In a recent meta-analysis, the risk of cervical cancer was 30% lower in women who used an IUD.[22]

ParaGard, a copper-containing IUD, is FDA-approved for up to 10 years of use. It has been shown to be effective for up to 20 years in some women.[23]

Mirena is FDA-approved for up to 5 years of use, but it has been shown to be effective for up to 7 years. It releases 20 mcg/day of levonorgestrel initially, which gradually decreases to 10 mcg/day over 5 years. *Mirena* is also approved for treatment of heavy menstrual bleeding.

Liletta is FDA-approved for up to 5 years of use. It releases 19.5 mcg/day of levonorgestrel initially, which gradually decreases to 9.8 mcg/day over 5 years. *Liletta* is the same size as *Mirena*.[24]

Skyla is FDA-approved for up to 3 years of use. It releases 14 mcg/day of levonorgestrel initially, which gradually decreases to 5 mcg/day over 3 years. *Skyla* is slightly smaller than *Mirena*, which may be advantageous in nulliparous women.

Kyleena is FDA-approved for up to 5 years of use. It releases 17.5 mcg/day of levonorgestrel initially, 9.8 mcg/day after 1 year, and 7.4 mcg/day after 5 years. *Kyleena* is the same size as *Skyla* and smaller than *Mirena* and *Liletta*.[25]

Adverse Effects – Uterine perforation occurs rarely during IUD placement. Bleeding and cramping are common during the first week. Irregular heavy bleeding and cramping may occur in the first 3-6 months after placement of the copper IUD. Irregular or light bleeding may occur during the first 3-6 months following insertion of a levonorgestrel IUD, but it generally decreases with continued use. The presence of an IUD does not increase the risk of a sexually transmitted infection (STI) or pelvic inflammatory disease (PID). Ovarian cysts have been reported with all levonorgestrel-releasing IUDs, but most are asymptomatic and resolve spontaneously. IUD expulsion can occur. Systemic levonorgestrel exposure is less with an IUD than with oral contraceptives, but adverse effects observed with oral formulations can occur.

BARRIER CONTRACEPTIVES — Barrier contraceptives have much higher failure rates than hormonal contraceptives or IUDs. Their effectiveness is highly user-dependent. Only condoms (not lamb intestine) prevent both pregnancy and STIs, including HIV infection.

Condoms – Both male and female (internal) condoms are available. Most **male** condoms in the US are made of latex; they are effective when used correctly, but can break when stored improperly or used with oil-based lubricants and vaginal medications. Alternatives for patients with latex sensitivity include lamb intestine and synthetic polyurethane condoms. Lamb intestine condoms do not protect against HIV and other viral infections. Synthetic polyurethane male condoms are more likely to break than latex condoms, and may be less effective in preventing pregnancy. **Female** condoms cover the external genitalia, possibly offering better protection against STIs, but they are less effective than male condoms. They can be used with either an oil- or water-based lubricant.

Diaphragms and Cervical Caps – Diaphragms and cervical caps are used with spermicide and placed over the cervix. Diaphragms can be placed up to 6 hours before intercourse and should not be removed for 6 hours afterward; they should not be left in place for more than 24 hours. Spermicide must be reapplied for each act of intercourse. *FemCap* should be placed 15-40 minutes before intercourse and should be left in place for at least 6 hours after intercourse (maximum 48 hours).

Spermicides – Nonoxynol-9, the only chemical spermicide available in the US, is marketed as a foam, film, gel, cream, suppository, and tablet. It must be placed in the vagina no more than one hour before intercourse and again before each act of intercourse. Suppositories, films, and tablets need to dissolve in order to be effective. Local irritation may occur.

Sponge – The *Today* sponge is an over-the-counter (OTC) barrier contraceptive containing the spermicide nonoxynol-9 that is moistened with water and placed over the cervix before intercourse. It is effective immediately after insertion and, if left in place, intercourse may be repeated for up to 24 hours. The sponge should not be removed for 6 hours after intercourse. It should be removed after 24-30 hours because of the risk of toxic shock syndrome. Sponges have been inferior to diaphragms in both effectiveness and user continuation rates.

FERTILITY AWARENESS-BASED METHODS — Fertility awareness-based methods of contraception involve periods of abstinence or use of barrier methods during the presumed fertile days of the menstrual cycle. These methods rely on observation of changes in cervical secretions and body temperature and estimation of the range of fertile days in the woman's usual menstrual cycle. Typical-use failure rates with these methods are high.

Natural Cycles, a fertility awareness-based mobile application (app), has recently been approved by the FDA. Based on information about a woman's menstrual cycle and daily morning basal temperature, the app predicts when she is most likely to be fertile and recommends barrier contraception or abstinence during this time. Other ovulation-prediction mobile apps are available, but they have not been approved by the FDA.

EMERGENCY CONTRACEPTION

IUD — A copper IUD inserted within 5 days after intercourse is the most effective method of emergency contraception (not an FDA-approved use); some studies indicate that it may also be effective if placed within 10 days after intercourse.[26,27] Heavy bleeding and cramping can occur in the first 3-6 months following insertion.

HORMONAL METHODS — Hormonal methods of emergency contraception, which can prevent or delay ovulation, can prevent 50-80% of pregnancies.[28] They are unlikely to be effective if taken just before or after ovulation.

Antiprogestin ECPs — Available only by prescription, ulipristal acetate *(Ella)* is the most effective hormonal option for emergency contraception. It is FDA-approved as an emergency contraceptive that can be taken up to 5 days after unprotected intercourse. Ulipristal acetate should be considered a first-line hormonal option for emergency contraception, especially for overweight or obese women.[29]

Progestin-Only ECPs — Single-dose levonorgestrel 1.5 mg is available over the counter for emergency contraception with no age restrictions. The dose should be taken as soon as possible (within 72 hours) after

Table 3. Some Emergency Contraceptives

Drug	Usual Dosage	Cost[1]
Ulipristal acetate –	30 mg PO once[3]	
Ella (Afaxys)[2]		$35.80
Levonorgestrel –	1.5 mg PO once[5]	
EContra One-Step (Afaxys)[4]		21.00[6]
My Way (Lupin)[4]		29.30
New Day (NorthStar)[4]		27.00
Option 2 (Perrigo)[4]		40.00[7]
Plan B One-Step (Foundation Consumer Healthcare)[4]		32.50
Preventeza (Combe)[4]		47.00[8]
Take Action (Teva Women's)[4]		26.30

1. Approximate WAC for one tablet. WAC = wholesaler acquisition cost, or manufacturer's published price to wholesalers; WAC represents published catalogue or list prices and may not represent an actual transactional price. Source: AnalySource® Monthly. September 5, 2018. Reprinted with permission by First Databank, Inc. All rights reserved. ©2018. www.fdbhealth.com/policies/drug-pricing-policy.
2. Available only by prescription.
3. Taken within 120 hours after unprotected intercourse or contraceptive failure.
4. Available over the counter with no age restriction.
5. Taken within 72 hours after unprotected intercourse or contraceptive failure.
6. Approximate retail cost according to the manufacturer.
7. Approximate cost at www.riteaid.com. Accessed September 27, 2018.
8. Cost for two single-dose packages according to the manufacturer.

unprotected intercourse or contraceptive failure. Some studies indicate that it may be effective if taken within 5 days.[30,31] The efficacy of single-dose levonorgestrel is significantly reduced in over-weight women.[26]

Combined ECPs – Standard combination oral contraceptives, taken in 2 doses 12 hours apart as soon as possible (within 72 hours) after unprotected intercourse, can be used for emergency contraception. They are less effective than single-dose levonorgestrel and multiple tablets are needed to achieve the recommended dose.

Adverse Effects – Nausea and vomiting occur more frequently with estrogen-progestin combinations than with levonorgestrel alone. Headache, abdominal pain, and breast tenderness have been reported with all hormonal ECPs. There have been no reports of fetal malformations caused by unsuccessful use of hormones for emergency contraception.

Choice of Contraceptives

1. ARA Aiken and J Trussell. Recent advances in contraception. F1000Prime Rep 2014; 6:113.
2. J Trussell and ARA Aiken. Contraceptive efficacy. In: RA Hatcher et al. Contraceptive Technology: Twenty-first revised edition. New York, NY: Ayer Company Publishers 2018.
3. KM Curtis et al. U.S. medical eligibility criteria for contraceptive use, 2016. MMWR Recomm Rep 2016; 65:1.
4. MF Gallo et al. 20 µg versus >20 µg estrogen combined oral contraceptives for contraception. Cochrane Database Syst Rev 2013; 8:CD003989.
5. A Edelman et al. Continuous or extended cycle vs. cyclic use of combined hormonal contraceptives for contraception. Cochrane Database Syst Rev 2014; 7:CD004695.
6. L Iversen et al. Association between contemporary hormonal contraception and ovarian cancer in women of reproductive age in Denmark: prospective, nationwide cohort study. BMJ 2018; 362:k3609.
7. AR Brant et al. Non-contraceptive benefits of hormonal contraception: established benefits and new findings. Curr Obstet Gynecol Rep 2017; 6:109.
8. R Słopień et al. Use of oral contraceptives for management of acne vulgaris and hirsutism in women of reproductive and late reproductive age. Menopause Rev 2018; 17:1.
9. Three new oral contraceptives. Med Lett Drugs Ther 2006; 48:77.
10. MK Trivedi et al. A review of hormone-based therapies to treat adult acne vulgaris in women. Int J Womens Dermatol 2017; 3:44.
11. Y Vinogradova et al. Use of combined oral contraceptives and risk of venous thromboembolism: nested case-control studies using the QResearch and CPRD databases. BMJ 2015; 350:h2135.
12. C Oedingen et al. Systematic review and meta-analysis of the association of combined oral contraceptives on the risk of venous thromboembolism: the role of the progestogen type and estrogen dose. Thromb Res 2018; 165:68.
13. LS Mørch et al. Contemporary hormonal contraception and the risk of breast cancer. N Engl J Med 2017; 377:2228.
14. CW Skovlund et al. Association of hormonal contraception with depression. JAMA Psychiatry 2016; 73:1154.
15. FDA. Labeling for combined hormonal contraceptives: guidance for industry. December 2017. Available at www.fda.gov/downloads/drugs/guidancecomplianceregulatoryinformation/guidances/UCM590673.pdf. Accessed September 27, 2018.
16. KB Simmons et al. Drug interactions between non-rifamycin antibiotics and hormonal contraception: a systematic review. Am J Obstet Gynecol 2018; 218:88.
17. ACOG. Committee opinion No. 602: depot medroxyprogesterone acetate and bone effects. Obstet Gynecol 2014; 123:1398.
18. ACOG. Practice bulletin No. 186: long-acting reversible contraception: implants and intrauterine devices. Obstet Gynecol 2017; 130:e251.
19. In brief: etonogestrel (Nexplanon) contraceptive implant. Med Lett Drugs Ther 2012; 54:12.
20. KM Curtis and JF Peipert. Long-acting reversible contraception. N Engl J Med 2017; 376:461.
21. JP Wu et al. Long-acting reversible contraception - highly efficacious, safe, and underutilized. JAMA 2018; 320:397.
22. VK Cortessis et al. Intrauterine device use and cervical cancer risk: a systematic review and meta-analysis. Obstet Gynecol 2017; 130:1226.

23. I Sivin. Utility and drawbacks of continuous use of a copper T IUD for 20 years. Contraception 2007; 75(6 Suppl):S70.
24. Liletta - a third levonorgestrel-releasing IUD. Med Lett Drugs Ther 2015; 57:99.
25. Kyleena - another hormonal IUD. Med Lett Drugs Ther 2017; 59:38.
26. ACOG. Practice bulletin summary No. 152: emergency contraception. Obstet Gynecol 2015; 126:685.
27. ND Goldstuck and D Wildemeersch. Practical advice for emergency IUD contraception in young women. Obstet Gynecol Int 2015; 2015:986439.
28. DT Baird. Emergency contraception: how does it work? Reprod Biomed Online 2009; 18 Suppl 1:32.
29. A Glasier. The rationale for use of ulipristal acetate as first line in emergency contraception: biological and clinical evidence. Gynecol Endocrinol 2014; 30:688.
30. G Piaggio et al. Effect on pregnancy rates of the delay in the administration of levonorgestrel for emergency contraception: a combined analysis of four WHO trials. Contraception 2011; 84:35.
31. K Cleland et al. Emergency contraception review: evidence-based recommendations for clinicians. Clin Obstet Gynecol 2014; 57:741.

DRUGS FOR
GERD and Peptic Ulcer Disease

Original publication date – January 2018

Gastroesophageal Reflux Disease

Gastroesophageal reflux disease (GERD) is the most frequent GI condition encountered in the outpatient setting; it affects about 20% of the US population. Heartburn and regurgitation are the classic symptoms of GERD. Other symptoms include dyspepsia, chest pain, belching, dysphagia, and chronic cough. While GERD is generally a benign condition, complications such as strictures, bleeding, and Barrett's esophagus can occur. Patients with GERD often report a decrease in quality of life.[1]

Endoscopy is recommended to evaluate alarm symptoms such as dysphagia, GI bleeding, anemia, weight loss, and persistent vomiting. It is also recommended for patients at high risk for complications, including those who do not respond to a 4-8 week trial of a proton pump inhibitor (PPI) and men >50 years old with chronic GERD (>5 years) who have additional risk factors for Barrett's esophagus, such as obesity and hiatal hernia.[2,3]

LIFESTYLE MODIFICATION — Lifestyle modifications, including not lying down for at least 2 hours after eating or drinking and elevating the head of the bed, should be a component of GERD management.[4] Weight loss can improve GERD symptoms and should be recommended for all

> ### Recommendations for Treatment of GERD, PUD, and *Helicobacter pylori* Infection
>
> #### Gastroesophageal Reflux Disease (GERD)
>
> - Lifestyle modifications, including not lying down for at least 2 hours after eating or drinking, elevating the head of the bed, and weight loss in patients who are overweight or have recently gained weight, should be a component of management.
> - Antacid or H2-receptor antagonist (H2RA) therapy is recommended for patients with mild, infrequent symptoms.
> - A proton pump inhibitor (PPI) is recommended for patients with more frequent symptoms or erosive esophagitis.
> - PPIs are more effective than H2RAs in relieving symptoms of GERD and in healing erosive esophagitis.
> - All PPIs appear to be similarly effective in healing erosive esophagitis and providing symptom relief.
> - Addition of an H2RA as needed may be beneficial for patients who have break-through nocturnal symptoms.
>
> #### Peptic Ulcer Disease (PUD)
>
> - All patients with PUD should be treated with a PPI.
> - All PPIs appear to be similarly effective in healing ulcers.
> - If the underlying cause can be identified and eliminated, long-term PPI therapy may not be needed.
> - For patients with idiopathic ulcers, long-term PPI therapy is recommended.
>
> #### *Helicobacter pylori* Infection
>
> - Bismuth quadruple therapy or concomitant quadruple therapy is recommended for first-line treatment of *H. pylori* infection.
> - Patients should be tested for eradication ≥4 weeks after completion of therapy.

patients who are overweight or have recently gained weight.[5-7] Routine avoidance of foods that have been thought to trigger reflux, such as chocolate, caffeine, alcohol, and spicy foods, is no longer recommended.

ACID-SUPPRESSIVE THERAPY — Medications that suppress gastric acid are the standard treatment for GERD. The choice of drug depends on the severity and frequency of symptoms and the presence or absence of esophagitis. PPIs have been shown to decrease GERD symptoms and heal esophagitis more effectively than other acid-suppressing drugs, and are generally preferred. All PPIs appear to be similarly effective in healing erosive esophagitis and providing symptom relief.[8,9]

Patients with mild, infrequent GERD symptoms can be treated with an antacid or H2-receptor antagonist (H2RA) as needed. For patients whose symptoms are inadequately controlled on an antacid or H2RA and for those who have more severe or frequent symptoms, a PPI taken once daily for 8 weeks is recommended. Patients who continue to have symptoms may benefit from twice-daily dosing or switching to another PPI.[8] Addition of an H2RA as needed at bedtime may be helpful for those who still have nocturnal symptoms despite twice-daily PPI therapy. Patients who have recurrent symptoms after stopping a PPI may respond to another course of treatment or to on-demand PPI therapy.

Treatment with a PPI for 8 weeks is recommended for healing of erosive esophagitis. Almost all patients with erosive esophagitis will have a relapse of symptoms within 6 months of stopping the PPI and most will require long-term maintenance therapy. Patients with Barrett's esophagus are generally treated with a PPI indefinitely.

PREGNANCY — Heartburn occurs in approximately 40-80% of pregnancies, and is largely attributed to a progesterone-mediated decrease in lower esophageal sphincter tone. Lifestyle modifications (not lying down for at least 2 hours after eating or drinking and elevating the head of the bed) can be helpful. Antacids can be tried for symptomatic relief, but products containing sodium bicarbonate or magnesium trisilate should be avoided. Sucralfate can be tried if antacids fail to relieve symptoms.[10]

An H2RA can be used if needed.[11] If symptoms persist on an H2RA, a PPI can be considered. PPIs are generally considered safe during pregnancy, but clinical data are limited. In a meta-analysis of 7 observational studies, there was no increase in the risk of congenital malformations with first-trimester PPI use (predominantly omeprazole).[12] A cohort study produced similar findings.[13]

Peptic Ulcer Disease

Helicobacter pylori infection is the most common cause of peptic ulcer disease (PUD). Use of nonsteroidal anti-inflammatory drugs (NSAIDs), including aspirin, is another common cause.

All patients with PUD should be treated with a PPI for ulcer healing. All PPIs appear to be similarly effective for this indication. If the underlying cause of PUD is identified and addressed (stopping the NSAID or eradicating *H. pylori* [see pages 77-85]), long-term antisecretory therapy may not be needed. Long-term PPI treatment is recommended for patients with idiopathic peptic ulcers, patients who develop PUD while taking low-dose aspirin for secondary prevention of cardiovascular disease, and those with NSAID-induced PUD who are unable to stop taking NSAIDs.[14]

Drugs for GERD and PUD

ANTACIDS — Antacids containing aluminum, magnesium, and/or calcium carbonate can provide rapid, but transient, relief of GERD and PUD symptoms. Aluminum and calcium carbonate can cause constipation, and magnesium-based antacids can cause diarrhea. Antacids can decrease the absorption of some other drugs by altering gastric acidity or by binding to other drugs in the GI tract.

H2-RECEPTOR ANTAGONISTS (H2RAs) — H2RAs inhibit the action of histamine at the H2 receptor of parietal cells, decreasing basal acid secretion and, to a lesser extent, food-stimulated acid secretion. All H2RAs are similarly effective for treatment of GERD and PUD. H2RAs have a faster onset of action than PPIs, but they are less effective than PPIs in relieving heartburn and healing erosive esophagitis,[8,15] and tolerance can develop quickly with continuous use. An H2RA can be used as needed for patients who have breakthrough nocturnal symptoms while taking a PPI.

Adverse Effects – Severe adverse effects are uncommon with H2RAs. Hepatitis, hematologic toxicity, and CNS effects such as headache, lethargy, depression, and cognitive impairment have occurred. Long-term use of an H2RA has been associated with vitamin B12 deficiency.[16] Cimetidine is weakly antiandrogenic and chronic use may rarely cause reversible impotence and gynecomastia.

Drug Interactions – H2RAs can decrease serum concentrations of drugs that require gastric acidity for absorption, such as itraconazole (*Sporanox*, and others) and the antiretroviral agents rilpivirine *(Edurant)* and atazanavir (*Reyataz*, and generics).

Cimetidine is a moderate inhibitor of CYP1A2, 2C19, and 2D6; it can increase serum concentrations of drugs that are metabolized by these enzymes, such as theophylline (*Theo-Dur*, and others), warfarin (*Coumadin*, and others), phenytoin (*Dilantin*, and others), and lidocaine (*Xylocaine*, and others).[17] Ranitidine, famotidine, and nizatidine are less likely to affect the hepatic metabolism of other drugs.

PROTON PUMP INHIBITORS (PPIs) — PPIs bind to the activated proton pump on the apical membrane of parietal cells, resulting in potent inhibition of acid secretion into the gastric lumen. They are more potent inhibitors of 24-hour acid secretion and heal peptic ulcers more rapidly than H2RAs.[15] PPIs are also more effective than H2RAs in relieving symptoms of GERD and in healing erosive esophagitis. All PPIs appear to be similarly effective in promoting mucosal healing and providing symptom relief.[18,19] Patients who do not respond to one PPI may respond to another.

PPIs have short serum half-lives, but their duration of action is longer than that of H2RAs, allowing for once-daily dosing in most patients. Since they require the presence of acid for activation, PPIs are most effective when taken on an empty stomach, 30-60 minutes before a meal. Other antisecretory drugs such as H2RAs should not be taken at the same

71

Table 1. Some Drugs for GERD and Peptic Ulcer Disease

Drug	Some Available Formulations
H2-Receptor Antagonists (H2RAs)	
Cimetidine – generic	200, 300, 400, 800 mg tabs; 300 mg/5 mL oral soln
Tagamet HB (OTC)[4] (Medtech)	200 mg tabs
Famotidine[5] – generic	20, 40 mg tabs; 10 mg/mL soln for inj; 40 mg/5 mL oral susp
Pepcid (Valeant)	20, 40 mg tabs; 40 mg/5 mL oral susp[6]
Pepcid AC (OTC)[4] (McNeil)	10, 20 mg tabs
Nizatidine – generic	150, 300 mg caps; 15 mg/mL oral soln
Ranitidine – generic	150, 300 mg tabs, caps; 25 mg/mL soln for inj; 15 mg/mL oral syrup
Zantac (GSK)	150, 300 mg tabs; 25 mg/mL soln for inj[8]; 15 mg/mL oral syrup
Zantac (OTC)[4] (Sanofi)	75, 150 mg tabs
Proton Pump Inhibitors (PPIs)[10]	
Dexlansoprazole – *Dexilant* (Takeda)	30, 60 mg delayed-release caps[11]
Esomeprazole magnesium[12] – generic	20, 40 mg delayed-release caps[11]
Nexium (AstraZeneca)	20, 40 mg delayed-release caps[11]; 2.5, 5, 10, 20, 40 mg powder for delayed-release susp
Nexium 24HR (OTC)[4] (Pfizer)	20 mg delayed-release caps, tabs
Esomeprazole sodium – generic	20, 40 mg vial for inj
Nexium IV	40 mg vial for inj
Lansoprazole[15] – generic	15, 30 mg delayed-release caps[11]; 15, 30 mg ODTs
Prevacid (Takeda)	
Prevacid 24HR (OTC)[4] (GSK)	15 mg delayed-release caps

ODTs = orally disintegrating tablets; OTC = over the counter
1. The lower end of the range is generally used for initial treatment of GERD. Higher or more frequent doses may be needed for patients with erosive esophagitis, peptic ulcer disease, hypersecretory conditions such as Zollinger-Ellison syndrome, or for treatment of *H. pylori* infection. NICE Clinical guideline [CG184]. 2014. Available at: www.nice.org.uk/guidance/cg184/chapter/Appendix-A-Dosage-information-on-proton-pump-inhibitors. Accessed January 4, 2018.
2. Approximate WAC for 30 days' treatment with the lowest usual oral dosage. WAC = wholesaler acquisition cost or manufacturer's published price to wholesalers; WAC represents a published catalogue or list price and may not represent an actual transactional price. Source: AnalySource® Monthly. December 5, 2017. Reprinted with permission by First Databank, Inc. All rights reserved. ©2017. www.fdbhealth.com/policies/drug-pricing-policy.
3. Taking the total daily dose at once in the evening may also be effective.
4. Also available generically.
5. Also available in combination with ibuprofen (*Duexis*).
6. *Pepcid* oral suspension is manufactured by Salix.

Usual Adult Dosage[1]	Cost[2]
200-400 mg bid[3]	$11.20
	16.30
20-40 mg bid[3]	5.70
	556.40
	15.10[7]
150 mg bid[3]	60.00
150 mg bid[3]	9.40
	361.90
	21.00[9]
30-60 mg once/d	258.70
20-40 mg once/d	96.30
	250.90
	16.40[13]
20-40 mg once/d	34.90[14]
	44.70[14]
15-30 mg once/d	63.60
	415.10
	18.50[13]

7. Approximate WAC for fifty 20-mg tablets.
8. *Zantac* solution for injection is manufactured by Teligent.
9. Approximate cost for forty-eight 150-mg tablets at cvs.com.
10. PPIs are generally taken 30-60 minutes before the first meal of the day. Taking one dose before the evening meal or taking the drug twice daily may be more effective for nocturnal acid control. PPIs should generally be swallowed whole and should not be crushed or chewed. Dexlansoprazole *(Dexilant)* can be taken with or without food. Omeprazole/sodium bicarbonate *(Zegerid)* should be taken on an empty stomach at least 1 hour before a meal.
11. Capsules can be opened and their contents sprinkled on soft food such as applesauce and consumed immediately.
12. Also available in combination with naproxen *(Vimovo, and generics)*.
13. Cost for 28 capsules or tablets.
14. Approximate WAC for one 40-mg vial.
15. Also available in combination with amoxicillin/clarithromycin *(Prevpac, and generics)* and in combination with naproxen *(Prevacid Naprapac)*.

Continued on next page

Drugs for GERD and Peptic Ulcer Disease

Table 1. Some Drugs for GERD and Peptic Ulcer Disease (continued)	
Drug	**Some Available Formulations**
Proton Pump Inhibitors (PPIs)[10] (continued)	
Omeprazole[16] – generic	10, 20, 40 mg delayed-release caps[11]
Prilosec (Covis)	2.5, 10 mg powder for delayed-release susp
Prilosec OTC[4] (AstraZeneca/P&G)	20 mg delayed-release tabs
Omeprazole/sodium bicarbonate[17] – generic	20/1680, 40/1680 mg/packet for susp; 20 mg/1.1 g, 40 mg/1.1 g caps[18]
Zegerid (Salix)[17]	
Zegerid OTC[4] (Bayer)[17]	20 mg/1.1 g, 40 mg/1.1 g caps[18]
Pantoprazole – generic	20, 40 mg delayed-release tabs; 40 mg vial for inj
Protonix (Pfizer)	20, 40 mg delayed-release tabs; 40 mg delayed-release granules for susp; 40 mg vial for inj
Rabeprazole – generic	20 mg delayed-release tabs
Aciphex (Eisai)	
Aciphex Sprinkle (Avadel)	5, 10 mg delayed-release sprinkle caps[19]
Others	
Misoprostol[21,22] – generic	100, 200 mcg tabs
Cytotec (Pfizer)	
Sucralfate[23] – generic	1 g tabs; 1 g/10 mL oral susp
Carafate (Aptalis)	

16. Also available in combination with amoxicillin/clarithromycin and with aspirin *(Yosprala)*.
17. Immediate-release formulation of omeprazole. Should be used with caution in patients on a low-sodium diet.
18. Since each capsule contains 1.1 g of sodium bicarbonate, two 20-mg capsules are not equivalent to one 40-mg capsule.

time as a PPI. Unlike H2RAs, tolerance to PPIs does not occur with continuous use.

PPIs are metabolized partially by CYP2C19. Patients who are CYP2C19 rapid metabolizers may have a decreased response to PPI treatment.[20,21]

Adverse Effects – PPIs are generally well tolerated. Headache, nausea, abdominal pain, constipation, flatulence, and diarrhea can

Usual Adult Dosage[1]	Cost[2]
20-40 mg once/d	$11.70
	529.10
	16.80[13]
20-40 mg once/d	
	2620.90
	3033.80
	16.10[13]
40 mg once/d	4.80
	393.30
20 mg once/d	44.50
	524.70
	490.10[20]
200 mcg bid or tid or qid	67.60
	307.20
1 g qid	33.70
	388.80

19. Contents of capsule should be sprinkled on soft food or liquid and taken within 15 minutes.
20. Approximate WAC for thirty 5-mg sprinkle capsules.
21. FDA-approved only for prevention of NSAID-induced gastric ulcers.
22. Also available in combination with diclofenac (*Arthrotec*, and generics).
23. FDA-approved only for short-term treatment and maintenance therapy of duodenal ulcers.

occur. Gynecomastia, hepatic failure, subacute myopathy, arthralgia, severe rash, and acute interstitial nephritis have been reported.

Observational studies have suggested that long-term PPI use is associated with a number of safety concerns, including fractures, dementia, *Clostridium difficile* infection, hypomagnesemia, vitamin B12 deficiency, chronic kidney disease, and increased all-cause mortality.[22-24] Most of these concerns are not supported by a causal mechanism or consistent data. The FDA has issued safety warnings regarding long-term PPI use and hypomagnesemia, fracture risk, and *Clostridium difficile*-associated diarrhea. The benefits of PPI treatment generally outweigh the risks in patients with a clear indication for long-term treatment.[25]

Drug Interactions – PPIs may decrease serum concentrations of drugs that require gastric acidity for absorption, such as itraconazole and the antiretroviral agents rilpivirine and atazanavir.

The PPIs omeprazole and esomeprazole are moderate inhibitors of CYP2C19 and could increase serum concentrations of drugs metabolized by this pathway, such as diazepam (*Valium*, and others) and phenytoin. Among the PPIs, omeprazole and esomeprazole appear to be the strongest inhibitors of CYP2C19 and pantoprazole appears to be the weakest.[26] The antiplatelet drug clopidogrel (*Plavix*, and generics) is converted to its active form by CYP2C19; inhibition of CYP2C19 may interfere with its activation. Whether concurrent use of clopidogrel and a PPI results in clinically significant adverse cardiovascular outcomes is not clear.[27,28] Since omeprazole and esomeprazole appear to be most likely to affect the antiplatelet activity of clopidogrel and the FDA specifically warns against their concomitant use, it would be reasonable to choose another PPI in patients taking clopidogrel.[29]

SUCRALFATE — An aluminum hydroxide complex of sucrose thought to act locally to protect ulcers from exposure to pepsin and gastric acid, sucralfate (*Carafate*, and generics) has been used to heal peptic ulcers and as maintenance treatment to prevent recurrence. It may not be effective in relieving ulcer pain, must be taken multiple times per day, and can reduce the absorption of drugs taken concomitantly.

Adverse Effects – Sucralfate is generally well tolerated, but it can cause constipation and aluminum toxicity, particularly in patients with renal impairment.

Drug Interactions – Sucralfate decreases the absorption of many other drugs, including fluoroquinolones, tetracyclines, and levothyroxine; administration should be separated by at least 2 hours.

ALGINATE — A polysaccharide derived from brown algae, alginate forms a floating foam/gel that acts as a physical barrier between the gastric contents and the gastroesophageal junction. In one randomized, placebo-controlled trial, addition of an alginate-based product (*Gaviscon Advance*; not available in the US) improved reflux symptoms in patients who had heartburn or regurgitation despite standard-dose PPI treatment.[30] In the US, *Gaviscon* products contain aluminum hydroxide and magnesium carbonate; sodium alginate is listed as an inactive ingredient. *Gaviscon Advance* and other products available outside the US contain larger amounts of alginate.

MISOPROSTOL — Misoprostol (*Cytotec*, and generics), a prostaglandin E1 analog, can prevent gastroduodenal ulcers in patients taking NSAIDs chronically, but it requires multiple daily doses and is not well tolerated.

Adverse Effects – Abdominal pain and dose-related diarrhea are the most common adverse effects of misoprostol. Severe nausea, constipation, dyspepsia, and flatulence can also occur. Misoprostol is an abortifacient and should not be used in women who are or could become pregnant.

Helicobacter pylori Infection

H. pylori is the most common cause of peptic ulcers[31]; eradication can promote gastric healing and prevent recurrence of gastric or duodenal ulcers.[32]

TESTING — Urea Breath Tests – A urea breath test can be used for office-based diagnosis of *H. pylori* infection. These tests typically have

Table 2. Preferred Regimens for *Helicobacter pylori* Infection[1]	
Drug	**Usual Adult Dosage**
Bismuth Quadruple Therapy	
Bismuth subsalicylate[4] (*Pepto-Bismol*, and others)	262 or 525 mg qid
+ metronidazole[7] (*Flagyl*, and others)	500 mg tid-qid
+ tetracycline[8] (*Sumycin*, and others)	500 mg qid
+ a PPI	See footnote 9
Concomitant Quadruple Therapy	
Clarithromycin[12] (*Biaxin*, and others)	500 mg bid
+ amoxicillin (*Amoxil*, and others)	1 g bid
+ metronidazole[7]	500 mg bid
+ a PPI	See footnote 9
Triple Therapy	
Clarithromycin[12]	500 mg bid
+ amoxicillin	1 g bid
+ a PPI	See footnote 9
or	
Clarithromycin[12]	500 mg bid
+ metronidazole	500 mg tid
+ a PPI	See footnote 9

PPI = proton pump inhibitor
1. Adapted from WD Chey et al. Am J Gastroenterol 2017; 112:212.
2. The PPI may be needed for a longer duration to heal the ulcer.
3. Approximate WAC for the regimen based on 14 days' treatment with the generic products at the lowest usual adult dosage. PPI cost is for 28 tablets of *Prilosec OTC*. WAC = wholesaler acquisition cost or manufacturer's published price to wholesalers; WAC represents a published catalogue or list price and may not represent an actual transactional price. Source: AnalySource® Monthly. December 5, 2017. Reprinted with permission by First Databank, Inc. All rights reserved. ©2018. www.fdbhealth.com/policies/drug-pricing-policy. Cost for bismuth subsalicylate is for 60 chewable tablets of *Pepto-Bismol* at cvs.com. Accessed January 4, 2018.
4. Or bismuth subcitrate 120-300 mg.
5. 14 days is recommended in areas with high metronidazole resistance (P Malfertheiner et al. Gut 2017; 66:6). In one study of US veterans in Houston, Texas, the prevalence of *H. pylori* resistance to metronidazole was 20.3% (S Shiota et al. Clin Gastroenterol Hepatol 2015; 13:1616).
6. Cost for 14 days' treatment if generic tetracycline is used. If the fixed-dose combination of bismuth subcitrate potassium/metronidazole/tetracycline (*Pylera*) is used, the cost is $819.10.

>90% sensitivity and specificity, and results are available within 10-20 minutes, but they require use of a mass spectrophotometer.[33]

Stool Antigen Tests – Stool antigen enzyme immunoassay (EIA) testing also has sensitivity and specificity >90%. It does not require special equipment and may be cheaper than urea breath tests.[34]

Duration[2]	Comments	Cost[3]
10-14 days[5]	▸ A preferred first-line option	$731.80[6]
10-14 days[5]	▸ A preferred first-line option	118.50[10]
14 days	▸ Should only be used in patients who reside in areas where clarithromycin resistance is <15% and in patients with no prior macrolide exposure for any indication[11]	97.40
		111.20

7. Or tinidazole (*Tindamax*, and generics) at the same dosage.
8. Generic tetracycline may not be available. The fixed-dose combination of bismuth subcitrate potassium/metronidazole/tetracycline *(Pylera)* can be used, but it is only packaged as a 10-day supply.
9. Standard oral PPI dosages are: esomeprazole 20 mg bid, lansoprazole 30 mg bid, omeprazole 20 mg bid, pantoprazole 40 mg bid, rabeprazole 20 mg bid. Some experts now recommend doubling the dose (e.g., omeprazole 40 mg bid). NICE Clinical Guideline [CG184]. 2014. Available at: www.nice.org.uk/guidance/cg184/chapter/Appendix-A-Dosage-information-on-proton-pump-inhibitors. Accessed January 4, 2018.
10. Cost is $966.00 for *Prevpac* or $573.70 for the generic version. *Prevpac* is supplied as 14 daily administration cards each containing two 30-mg lansoprazole capsules, four 500-mg amoxicillin capsules, and two 500-mg clarithromycin tablets.
11. Clarithromycin resistance rates are considered to be ≥15% unless local resistance patterns that show otherwise are available.
12. Clarithromycin may increase the risk of cardiac adverse effects and death in patients with coronary artery disease (FDA Drug Safety Communication, February 2018).

Serology – Serologic antibody tests for *H. pylori* lack specificity and sensitivity and do not differentiate between active and past infection. They can not be used for documenting *H. pylori* eradication.

Endoscopy with Biopsy – *H. pylori* can be diagnosed from endoscopic biopsies using urease testing or by histopathology. Urease testing of biopsy specimens has >90% sensitivity and specificity. Rapid tests are available that provide results in one hour. Histologic diagnosis from biopsy specimens has >95% sensitivity and specificity, but it takes longer and is more expensive than urease testing.

Drug Interference – The sensitivity of urea breath tests, stool antigen tests, and urease testing of biopsy specimens for *H. pylori* is reduced by use of PPIs, bismuth-containing products, and antibiotics. Patients should not take a PPI for at least 1-2 weeks or a bismuth-containing product or antibiotics for at least 4 weeks before these tests.

TREATMENT OF *H. PYLORI* – Preferred regimens for the treatment of *H. pylori* infection are listed in Table 2 and some alternative regimens are listed in Table 3.

In clinical trials, combinations of antimicrobial drugs have been successful in eradicating *H. pylori*, but in clinical practice, eradication rates have been reduced due to bacterial resistance and poor patient adherence to multi-drug regimens. Local resistance patterns and antibiotic susceptibility testing should guide the selection of antibacterial drugs, but they are not readily available in the US.

The efficacy of **clarithromycin triple therapy** (a PPI, clarithromycin, and amoxicillin or metronidazole) has diminished because of increasing clarithromycin resistance. This regimen should be used for first-line treatment only in patients who have no history of macrolide use for any indication and reside in areas where *H. pylori* resistance to clarithromycin is known to be <15%. Data on *H. pylori* resistance rates in the US are limited. Clarithromycin resistance rates in the US should be considered to be ≥15% unless local resistance patterns show otherwise. In a recent study performed in Houston, Texas, the prevalence of resistance to clarithromycin was 16.4%.[35]

Bismuth quadruple therapy (a PPI, bismuth, tetracycline, and metronidazole or tinidazole) and **concomitant quadruple therapy** (a PPI, clarithromycin, amoxicillin, and metronidazole or tinidazole) are more effective than clarithromycin triple therapy for eradication of *H. pylori* and are now recommended for first-line treatment of *H. pylori* infection.[36]

Some alternative regimens for treatment of *H. pylori* infection include **sequential therapy**, **levofloxacin sequential therapy**, **levofloxacin triple therapy**, and **hybrid therapy**.[37]

PPIs – Adequate acid suppression with PPIs is associated with higher *H. pylori* cure rates.[21] A higher intragastric pH improves antibiotic stability and bioavailability, resulting in higher concentrations.[38] It also promotes *H. pylori* replication making it more susceptible to antibiotic treatment.

The potency of PPIs in maintaining a higher gastric pH can vary from drug to drug.[39,40] One meta-analysis that included 35 studies suggested that *H. pylori* eradication rates were higher with esomeprazole or rabeprazole than with omeprazole, lansoprazole, or pantoprazole.[41]

All PPIs should be given twice daily for treatment of *H. pylori* infection. Some experts recommend using high PPI doses (e.g., omeprazole 40 mg bid), especially for patients who are CYP2C19 rapid metabolizers.[42]

TREATMENT FAILURE — Testing for eradication of *H. pylori* should be performed at least 4 weeks after completion of therapy. Patients should not use a PPI for 1-2 weeks before testing. Patients who are still infected should be treated with a different regimen. Bismuth quadruple therapy or levofloxacin triple therapy can be used for patients who initially received a regimen containing clarithromycin.[43-45] Those who were initially treated with bismuth quadruple therapy can be treated with concomitant quadruple therapy or levofloxacin triple therapy.

ADVERSE EFFECTS — Bismuth subsalicylate can temporarily turn the tongue and stool black and can cause tinnitus. The most common adverse effects associated with use of antibacterials for treatment of *H. pylori* are GI disturbances such as diarrhea, nausea, vomiting,

Table 3. Some Alternative Regimens for *Helicobacter pylori* Infection

Drug	Usual Adult Dosage
Sequential Therapy	
Amoxicillin (*Amoxil*, and others)	1 g bid
+ a PPI	See footnote 3
followed by	
clarithromycin[5] (*Biaxin*, and others)	500 mg bid
+ metronidazole[4] (*Flagyl*, and others)	500 mg bid
+ a PPI	See footnote 3
Levofloxacin Sequential Therapy	
Amoxicillin	1 g bid
+ a PPI	See footnote 3
followed by	
levofloxacin (*Levaquin*, and generics)	500 mg once/d
+ metronidazole[4]	500 mg bid
+ a PPI	See footnote 3
Hybrid Therapy	
Amoxicillin	1 g bid
+ a PPI	See footnote 3
followed by	
amoxicillin	1 g bid
+ clarithromycin[5]	500 mg bid
+ metronidazole[4]	500 mg bid
+ a PPI	See footnote 3
Levofloxacin Triple Therapy	
Levofloxacin	500 mg once/d
+ amoxicillin	1 g bid
+ a PPI	See footnote 3

PPI = proton pump inhibitor
1. The PPI may be needed for a longer duration to heal the ulcer.
2. Approximate WAC for the regimen based on 14 days' treatment with the generic products (except LOAD and rifabutin triple therapy, which are based on 10 days' treatment) at the lowest usual adult dosage. PPI cost is for 28 tablets of *Prilosec OTC*. WAC = wholesaler acquisition cost or manufacturer's published price to wholesalers; WAC represents a published catalogue or list price and may not represent an actual transactional price. Source: AnalySource® Monthly. December 5, 2017. Reprinted with permission by First Databank, Inc. All rights reserved. ©2017. www.fdbhealth.com/policies/drug-pricing-policy.

Duration[1]	Comments	Cost[2]
5-7 days	▸ May be less effective than concomitant quadruple therapy	$64.10
5-7 days		
5-7 days	▸ Levofloxacin resistance is a concern	38.60
5-7 days		
7 days	▸ US efficacy data are lacking	67.80
7 days		
10-14 days	▸ Levofloxacin resistance is a concern	46.50

3. Standard oral PPI dosages are: esomeprazole 20 mg bid, lansoprazole 30 mg bid, omeprazole 20 mg bid, pantoprazole 40 mg bid, rabeprazole 20 mg bid. Some experts now recommend doubling the dose (e.g., omeprazole 40 mg bid). NICE Clinical Guideline [CG184]. 2014. Available at: www.nice.org. uk/guidance/cg184/chapter/Appendix-A-Dosage-information-on-proton-pump-inhibitors. Accessed January 4, 2018. For high-dose dual therapy, the PPI should be given tid or qid.
4. Or tinidazole (*Tindamax*, and generics) at the same dosage.
5. Clarithromycin may increase the risk of cardiac adverse effects and death in patients with coronary artery disease (FDA Drug Safety Communication, February 2018).

Continued on next page

Table 3. Some Alternative Regimens for *Helicobacter pylori* Infection (continued)	
Drug	**Usual Adult Dosage**
Other Regimens	
Levofloxacin Quadruple Therapy (LOAD)	
Levofloxacin	250 mg once/d
+ omeprazole[6]	40 mg once/d
+ nitazoxanide *(Alinia)*	500 mg bid
+ doxycycline	100 mg once/d
Rifabutin Triple Therapy	
Rifabutin (*Mycobutin*, and generics)	300 mg once/d
+ amoxicillin	1 g bid
+ a PPI	See footnote 3
High-Dose Dual Therapy	
Amoxicillin	1 g tid or 750 mg qid
+ a PPI	See footnote 3
6. Or equivalent dose of another PPI.	

anorexia, and abdominal pain. Clarithromycin commonly causes taste disturbances that some patients find intolerable, and it can cause QT-interval prolongation. *Update 3/7/2018:* The FDA updated the labeling of clarithromycin (*Biaxin*, and others) to warn about an increased risk of adverse cardiac events and death in patients with coronary artery disease who were treated with the drug.[47] Metronidazole and tinidazole frequently cause a metallic taste and can cause a disulfiram-like reaction to alcohol; neurologic adverse effects, including seizures and neuropathy, have also been reported with use of these drugs, particularly at high doses.

DRUG INTERACTIONS — Clarithromycin is a strong inhibitor of CYP3A4 and P-glycoprotein (P-gp) and may increase serum concentrations of drugs that are metabolized by these pathways.[17] Taking clarithromycin with other drugs that prolong the QT interval, especially those metabolized by CYP3A4, can increase the risk of QT-interval prolongation and torsades de pointes.[46] Metronidazole is an inhibitor of

Duration[1]	Comments	Cost[2]
7-10 days	► One open-label trial reported an eradication rate of 90%	$1770.70
10 days	► Should only be used for salvage treatment ► Can cause myelotoxicity and may lead to development of resistant strains of *Mycobacterium tuberculosis*	309.70
14 days	► Can be considered for salvage treatment	27.70

CYP2C9 and may increase serum concentrations of drugs metabolized by this isozyme, including warfarin. Coadministration of antacids or products containing calcium, magnesium, or iron can decrease absorption of tetracycline and levofloxacin; it should be taken 2 hours before or 6 hours after these products.

1. JE Richter and JH Rubenstein. Presentation and epidemiology of gastroesophageal reflux disease. Gastroenterology 2017 Aug 3 (epub).
2. NJ Shaheen et al. Upper endoscopy for gastroesophageal reflux disease: best practice advice from the clinical guidelines committee of the American College of Physicians. Ann Intern Med 2012; 157:808.
3. ASGE Standards of Practice Committee. The role of endoscopy in the management of GERD. Gastrointest Endosc 2015; 81:1305.
4. E Ness-Jensen et al. Lifestyle intervention in gastroesophageal reflux disease. Clin Gastroenterol Hepatol 2016; 14:175.
5. M Singh et al. Weight loss can lead to resolution of gastroesophageal reflux disease symptoms: a prospective intervention trial. Obesity (Silver Spring) 2013; 21:284.
6. E Ness-Jensen et al. Weight loss and reduction in gastroesophageal reflux. A prospective population-based cohort study: the HUNT study. Am J Gastroenterol 2013; 108:376.

7. BC Jacobson et al. Body-mass index and symptoms of gastroesophageal reflux in women. N Engl J Med 2006; 354:2340.
8. PO Katz et al. Guidelines for the diagnosis and management of gastroesophageal reflux disease. Am J Gastroenterol 2013; 108:308.
9. KE Sigterman et al. Short-term treatment with proton pump inhibitors, H2-receptor antagonists and prokinetics for gastro-oesophageal reflux disease-like symptoms and endoscopy negative reflux disease. Cochrane Database Syst Rev 2013; 5:CD002095.
10. C Body and JA Christie. Gastrointestinal disease in pregnancy: nausea, vomiting, hyperemesis gravidum, gastroesophageal reflux disease, constipation, and diarrhea. Gastroenterol Clin North Am 2016; 45:267.
11. CJ van der Woude et al. Management of gastrointestinal and liver diseases during pregnancy. Gut 2014; 63:1014.
12. SK Gill et al. The safety of proton pump inhibitors (PPIs) in pregnancy: a meta-analysis. Am J Gastroenterol 2009; 104:1541.
13. B Pasternak and A Hviid. Use of proton-pump inhibitors in early pregnancy and the risk of birth defects. N Engl J Med 2010; 363:2114.
14. L Laine and DM Jensen. Management of patients with ulcer bleeding. Am J Gastroenterol 2012; 107:345.
15. U Dutta and P Moayyedi. Management of reflux-related symptoms. Best Pract Res Clin Gastroenterol 2013; 27:387.
16. JR Lam et al. Proton pump inhibitor and histamine 2 receptor antagonist use and vitamin B12 deficiency. JAMA 2013; 310:2435.
17. Inhibitors and inducers of CYP enzymes and P-glycoprotein. Med Lett Drugs Ther 2017 September 18 (epub). Available at: medicalletter.org/downloads/CYP_PGP_Tables.pdf. Accessed January 4, 2018.
18. YM Kung et al. Recent advances in the pharmacological management of gastroesophageal reflux disease. Dig Dis Sci 2017; 62:3298.
19. Which PPI? Med Lett Drugs Ther 2015; 57:91.
20. T Furuta et al. Influence of CYP2C19 pharmacogenetic polymorphism on proton pump inhibitor-based therapies. Drug Metab Pharmacokinet 2005; 20:153.
21. J Molina-Infante and A Shiotani. Practical aspects in choosing a *Helicobacter pylori* therapy. Gastroenterol Clin North Am 2015; 44:519.
22. Safety of long-term PPI use. Med Lett Drugs Ther 2017; 59:131.
23. MF Vaezi et al. Complications of proton pump inhibitor therapy. Gastroenterology 2017; 153:35.
24. SN Landi et al. No increase in risk of acute myocardial infarction in privately insured adults prescribed proton pump inhibitors vs histamine-2 receptor antagonists (2002-2014). Gastroenterology 2017 Nov 6 (epub).
25. DE Freedberg et al. The risks and benefits of long-term use of proton pump inhibitors: expert review and best practice advice from the American Gastroenterological Association. Gastroenterology 2017; 152:706.
26. RS Wedemeyer and H Blume. Pharmacokinetic drug interaction profiles of proton pump inhibitors: an update. Drug Saf 2014; 37:201.
27. SA Scott et al. Antiplatelet drug interactions with proton pump inhibitors. Expert Opin Drug Metab Toxicol 2014; 10:175.

28. SD Bouziana and K Tziomalos. Clinical relevance of clopidogrel-proton pump inhibitors interaction. World J Gastrointest Pharmacol Ther 2015; 6:17.

29. Drug interaction: clopidogrel and PPIs. Med Lett Drugs Ther 2017; 59:39.

30. C Reimer et al. Randomised clinical trial: alginate (Gaviscon Advance) vs. placebo as add-on therapy in reflux patients with inadequate response to a once daily proton pump inhibitor. Aliment Pharmacol Ther 2016; 43:899.

31. AC Ford et al. Eradication therapy for peptic ulcer disease in *Helicobacter pylori*-positive people. Cochrane Database Syst Rev 2016; 4:CD003840.

32. YC Lee et al. Association between *Helicobacter pylori* eradication and gastric cancer incidence: a systematic review and meta-analysis. Gastroenterology 2016; 150:1113.

33. MP Dore et al. Dyspepsia: when and how to test for *Helicobacter pylori* infection. Gastroenterol Res Pract 2016 April 28 (epub).

34. J Fashner and AC Gitu. Diagnosis and treatment of peptic ulcer disease and *H. pylori* infection. Am Fam Physician 2015; 91:236.

35. S Shiota et al. Antibiotic resistance of *Helicobacter pylori* among male United States veterans. Clin Gastroenterol Hepatol 2015; 13:1616.

36. WD Chey et al. ACG clinical guideline: treatment of *Helicobacter pylori* infection. Am J Gastroenterol 2017; 112:212.

37. Drugs for Helicobacter pylori infection. Med Lett Drugs Ther 2017; 59:113.

38. T Furuta and DY Graham. Pharmacologic aspects of eradication therapy for *Helicobacter pylori* infection. Gastroenterol Clin North Am 2010; 39:465.

39. J Kirchheiner et al. Relative potency of proton-pump inhibitors-comparison of effects on intragastric pH. Eur J Clin Pharmacol 2009; 65:19.

40. DY Graham and A Tansel. Interchangeable use of proton pump inhibitors based on relative potency. Clin Gastroenterol Hepatol 2017 Sep 28 (epub).

41. AG McNicholl et al. Meta-analysis: esomeprazole or rabeprazole vs. first-generation pump inhibitors in the treatment of *Helicobacter pylori* infection. Aliment Pharmacol Ther 2012; 36:414.

42. P Malfertheiner et al. Management of *Helicobacter pylori* infection–the Maastricht V/ Florence consensus report. Gut 2017; 66:6.

43. AC Marin et al. Efficacy of a second-line levofloxacin-containing triple therapy after the failure of the non-bismuth sequential or concomitant treatments: systematic review and meta-analysis. Helicobacter 2014; 19 (Suppl 1):139, abstract P11.39.

44. AC Marin et al. A review of rescue regimens after clarithromycin-containing triple therapy failure (for *Helicobacter pylori* eradication). Expert Opin Pharmacother 2013; 14:843.

45. T Shaikh and CA Fallone. Effectiveness of second through sixth line salvage *Helicobacter pylori* treatment: bismuth quadruple therapy is almost always a reasonable choice. Can J Gastroenterol Hepatol 2016 March 29 (epub).

46. RL Woosley and KA Romero. QT drugs list. Available at: www.crediblemeds.org. Accessed January 4, 2018.

47. FDA Drug Safety Communication: FDA review finds additional data supports the potential for increased long-term risks with antibiotic clarithromycin (Biaxin) in patients with heart disease. Available at: www.fda.gov/drugs/drugsafety/ucm597289.htm. Accessed March 7, 2018.

DRUGS FOR
Inflammatory Bowel Disease

Original publication date – July 2018

Management of both ulcerative colitis (UC) and Crohn's disease (CD) is based on disease severity. Disease location (proctitis, left-sided colitis, or extensive colitis) also plays a role in drug selection. Some drugs for induction and maintenance of remission of inflammatory bowel disease (IBD) are listed in Table 3.

AMINOSALICYLATES — Aminosalicylates (5-ASAs) are effective for induction and maintenance of remission in mild to moderate UC.[1,2] Sulfasalazine (*Azulfidine*, and generics) may also be effective for relief of symptoms in mild to moderate colonic CD, but it does not appear to be more effective than placebo in achieving mucosal healing and it is poorly tolerated.[3]

Formulations – Since 5-ASA is absorbed in the small intestine, oral formulations require delayed-release mechanisms to ensure the drug reaches the colon. *Pentasa* releases mesalamine gradually throughout the GI tract. Other mesalamine formulations delay release until the distal ileum and colon. Sulfasalazine, balsalazide (*Colazal*, and others), and olsalazine *(Dipentum)* are prodrugs; 5-ASA is azo-bonded to a second moiety and released in the colon following bacterial cleavage of the bond. Mesalamine is also available as an enema (*Rowasa*, and generics) and a rectal suppository *(Canasa)*.

Recommendations for Treatment of IBD
Ulcerative Colitis
▸ In mild to moderate disease, aminosalicylates are used as first-line therapy for both induction and maintenance of remission.
▸ In moderate to severe disease, corticosteroids, including extended-release budesonide, are used to induce remission when aminosalicylates are ineffective. Corticosteroids are not recommended for maintenance of remission.
▸ In moderate to severe disease, azathioprine or mercaptopurine is used for maintenance of remission.
▸ A TNF inhibitor (infliximab, adalimumab, or golimumab) can be used for induction and maintenance of remission in moderate to severe disease in patients who have not responded to other therapies or are corticosteroid-dependent.
▸ In moderate to severe disease, vedolizumab or tofacitinib may be used for induction and maintenance of remission when other drugs are ineffective or intolerable.
Crohn's Disease
▸ Corticosteroids, including ileal-release budesonide, can be used to induce remission. They are not recommended for maintenance of remission.
▸ For maintenance of remission in moderate to severe disease, azathioprine or mercaptopurine is used. Methotrexate is an alternative.
▸ In moderate to severe disease, a TNF inhibitor (infliximab, adalimumab, or certolizumab pegol) alone or in combination with azathioprine or mercaptopurine can be used for induction and maintenance of remission.
▸ In moderate to severe disease, ustekinumab or vedolizumab may be effective for induction and maintenance of remission when other drugs are ineffective or intolerable.

Efficacy – In mild to moderate UC, oral 5-ASAs induce remission in about 40% of patients and maintain remission for 6-12 months in about 60%.[4] In distal UC and proctitis, mesalamine suppositories or enemas may be more effective than oral formulations in inducing and maintaining remission. Combination therapy with oral and rectal mesalamine may be more effective than use of either formulation alone in distal UC.

Adverse Effects – The most common adverse effects of 5-ASAs are nausea, vomiting, diarrhea, headache, and abdominal pain. Pancreatitis, hepatotoxicity, pericarditis, pneumonitis, and a lupus-like syndrome have been reported. Nephrotoxicity can occur rarely. An acute intolerance syndrome that can mimic an exacerbation of UC can occur with mesalamine.

Drug Interactions – Coadministration with antacids could result in premature dissolution of the pH-sensitive coating of extended- and delayed-release mesalamine formulations. Theoretically, a similar interaction could occur with proton pump inhibitors (PPIs), such as omeprazole (*Prilosec*, and others), or with H2-receptor antagonists (H2RAs), such as ranitidine (*Zantac*, and others). Sulfasalazine may decrease the absorption of digoxin (*Lanoxin*, and generics).

5-ASAs inhibit thiopurine methyltransferase (TPMT) and may decrease the metabolism of azathioprine and 6-MP, which could increase their toxicity, especially in patients with inherited TPMT deficiency.

CORTICOSTEROIDS — Corticosteroids are effective for short-term symptom control and induction of remission in acute UC and CD. They are used systemically only for suppression of acute inflammation, and are then tapered and stopped. They should not be used in the presence of abscess or fistula.

Efficacy – In one retrospective study in 146 patients, 51% of patients with UC and 40% of those with CD had a complete response to corticosteroid treatment at 30 days; 31% and 35%, respectively, had a partial response.[5] Most patients whose IBD responds to corticosteroid treatment will relapse without maintenance therapy.

Adverse Effects – Corticosteroids can increase the risk of infection and cause fluid retention, osteoporosis, osteonecrosis, cataracts, glaucoma, impaired skin healing, acne, hirsutism, insomnia, mood disorders, Cushing's syndrome, weight gain, hyperglycemia, and hypothalamic-pituitary-adrenal (HPA) axis suppression.

Drugs for Inflammatory Bowel Disease

Table 1. Drugs for Ulcerative Colitis	
Recommended Drugs	**Some Alternatives**
Mild to Moderate	
Induction of Remission	
Mesalamine (oral, rectal)	Budesonide
Balsalazide	Prednisone
Olsalazine	Sulfasalazine
Hydrocortisone (rectal)	Infliximab
Budesonide (rectal)	Adalimumab
	Golimumab
	Vedolizumab
Maintenance of Remission	
Mesalamine (oral, rectal)	Azathioprine
Balsalazide	Mercaptopurine
Olsalazine	Sulfasalazine
	Infliximab
	Adalimumab
	Golimumab
	Vedolizumab
Moderate to Severe	
Induction of Remission	
Prednisone	Infliximab
Hydrocortisone	Adalimumab
Methylprednisolone	Golimumab
	Cyclosporine
	Tacrolimus
	Vedolizumab
	Tofacitinib
Maintenance of Remission	
Azathioprine	Sulfasalazine
Mercaptopurine	Golimumab
Infliximab	Vedolizumab
Adalimumab	Tofacitinib

Continued on next page

Rectal Corticosteroids – Rectally administered corticosteroids are effective for treatment of distal UC. Enemas can reach the splenic flexure, while foams only reach the distal part of the sigmoid colon.

Table 1. Drugs for Ulcerative Colitis (continued)	
Recommended Drugs	**Some Alternatives**
Pouchitis	
Induction of Remission	
Ciprofloxacin	Rifaximin
Metronidazole	Budesonide
	Infliximab
Maintenance of Remission	
Probiotics (*VSL #3*)	Mesalamine (rectal)
Metronidazole	Infliximab
Ciprofloxacin	
Rifaximin	

Budesonide – Budesonide is a synthetic corticosteroid with a strong affinity for glucocorticoid receptors and a high ratio of topical to systemic anti-inflammatory effects. An oral extended-release formulation of budesonide *(Uceris)* that distributes the drug throughout the colon is FDA-approved for induction of remission in mild to moderate UC. In patients with active mild to moderate UC, remission rates were higher with *Uceris* (18%) than with oral mesalamine (12%).[6] *Uceris* rectal foam has been modestly effective in inducing remission in patients with moderate to severe distal UC.[7]

Budesonide is also available orally in an ileal-release formulation (*Entocort EC*, and generics) for induction of remission in mild to moderate CD of the ileum and/or ascending colon. Guidelines recommend against using the drug for more than 4 months to maintain remission of CD.[3]

Budesonide causes less short-term corticosteroid toxicity than prednisone; whether it is safer in the long term is not clear. Abnormal adrenocorticoid stimulation tests and bone density changes can occur with budesonide.

Budesonide is a CYP3A4 substrate; concurrent administration with drugs that inhibit CYP3A4 could increase its toxicity.[8] Drugs that alter gastrointestinal pH (antacids, PPIs, H2RAs) may affect the release and absorption of oral budesonide.

THIOPURINES — **Azathioprine** (*Imuran*, and generics) and **mercaptopurine** (6-MP), its active metabolite, are effective in maintaining remission in both UC and CD. Since they can take 3-6 months to achieve maximal effect, they are used for long-term treatment and not for immediate suppression of active inflammation.

Efficacy – In controlled trials, azathioprine and 6-MP have been significantly more effective than placebo in maintaining remission in both UC and CD.[9,10]

With TNF Inhibitors – In a study in patients with moderate to severe CD who had not been previously treated with immunosuppressive or biologic therapy, the combination of azathioprine and the tumor necrosis factor (TNF) inhibitor infliximab (*Remicade*, and others) was more effective than either drug alone.[11] The results of another study suggest that the combination of infliximab and azathioprine is also more effective than either drug alone for treatment of UC.[12]

Adverse Effects – Azathioprine and 6-MP can cause myelosuppression and hepatotoxicity; complete blood counts and liver function tests should be monitored routinely during treatment. Patients with low TPMT activity are at increased risk for myelosuppression; TPMT testing should be considered before starting therapy. These drugs can also increase the risk of infection and cause nausea, vomiting, diarrhea, rash, pulmonary edema, pancreatitis, and hypersensitivity reactions. Use of thiopurines has been associated with an increase in the risk of non-melanoma skin cancer; the risk decreases after the drug is stopped.[13] Long-term thiopurine use has been associated with an increase in lymphoma risk; the risk appears to be greatest when taken in combination with TNF inhibitors.[14] Hepatosplenic T-cell lymphoma has been reported in patients taking azathioprine or 6-MP, both alone and in combination with a TNF inhibitor.

Table 2. Drugs for Crohn's Disease	
Recommended Drugs	**Some Alternatives**
Mild to Moderate	
Induction of Remission	
Budesonide	Prednisone
	Metronidazole
	Ciprofloxacin
	Rifaximin
Maintenance of Remission	
Azathioprine	Budesonide
Mercaptopurine	Methotrexate
Moderate to Severe	
Induction of Remission	
Prednisone	Vedolizumab
Methylprednisolone	Natalizumab
Infliximab	Ustekinumab
Adalimumab	
Certolizumab pegol	
Maintenance of Remission	
Infliximab	Methotrexate
Adalimumab	Vedolizumab
Certolizumab pegol	Natalizumab
Azathioprine	Ustekinumab
Mercaptopurine	
Perianal and Fistulizing Disease	
Induction of Remission	
Metronidazole ± Ciprofloxacin	
Infliximab	
Maintenance of Remission	
Azathioprine	
Mercaptopurine	
Infliximab	

Drug Interactions – Allopurinol (*Zyloprim*, and generics) and febuxostat (*Uloric*) inhibit azathioprine and 6-MP metabolism by xanthine oxidase, increasing their toxicity; the dose of azathioprine or 6-MP should be reduced if allopurinol is used concurrently, and concomitant use of febuxostat is contraindicated. (In some patients who are intolerant or refractory to thiopurine therapy, addition of allopurinol to a low-dose thiopurine can increase efficacy and reduce toxicity.[15]) Mesalamine inhibits TPMT and may decrease the metabolism of azathioprine and 6-MP, which could increase their toxicity, especially in patients with inherited TPMT deficiency.

Concurrent use of a thiopurine and an angiotensin-converting enzyme (ACE) inhibitor or trimethoprim/sulfamethoxazole (*Bactrim*, and others) can cause severe leukopenia. Azathioprine and 6-MP may decrease the anticoagulant effect of warfarin (*Coumadin*, and others).

METHOTREXATE — In CD, methotrexate can be used as an alternative to azathioprine or 6-MP to maintain remission and permit withdrawal of corticosteroids. It has not been clearly shown to be effective in UC.

Efficacy – Several studies have found intramuscular methotrexate effective in maintaining remission in patients with CD. It may also be effective in inducing remission in steroid-refractory CD.[16] In one study, however, addition of subcutaneous methotrexate to infliximab was no more effective in maintaining remission than infliximab alone.[17]

Adverse Effects – Methotrexate can cause myelosuppression, alopecia, rash, stomatitis, vomiting, diarrhea, GI hemorrhage, hepatotoxicity, renal failure, interstitial pneumonia, toxic epidermal necrolysis, Stevens-Johnson syndrome, hypotension, blurred vision, headache, nephropathy, and hyperuricemia. Supplementation with folic acid may reduce methotrexate toxicity.

Drug Interactions – Trimethoprim and other drugs that interfere with folate metabolism may increase bone marrow suppression caused by methotrexate. PPIs and drugs that reduce renal function, particularly NSAIDs, may increase serum concentrations of methotrexate and possibly its toxicity.

CYCLOSPORINE — The calcineurin inhibitor cyclosporine (*Sandimmune*, and others) is used as rescue therapy to avoid colectomy in patients with severe steroid-resistant UC. Cyclosporine has not been found to be effective in CD.

Efficacy – In a retrospective cohort study in patients with acute severe steroid-refractory UC, cyclosporine and infliximab appeared to be similarly effective in preventing colectomy at one and five years.[18]

Adverse Effects – Cyclosporine can increase the risk of infection and cause diarrhea, nausea, vomiting, and gingival hyperplasia, pruritus, headache, seizures, tremors, visual disturbances, hypertension, hepatotoxicity, nephrotoxicity, paresthesias, and anaphylaxis.

Drug Interactions – Nephrotoxic effects may be additive when cyclosporine is used with other nephrotoxic drugs such as aminoglycosides. Concurrent use of potassium-sparing diuretics such as spironolactone (*Aldactone*, and generics) may increase the risk of hyperkalemia. Cyclosporine is both a substrate and an inhibitor of CYP3A4 and P-glycoprotein; use with CYP3A4 inhibitors may increase its toxicity and use with CYP3A4 inducers may decrease its effectiveness.[8]

TNF INHIBITORS — Three tumor necrosis factor (TNF) inhibitors – infliximab *(Remicade)*, adalimumab *(Humira)*, and golimumab *(Simponi)* – are FDA-approved for treatment of moderate to severe UC refractory to conventional therapies.[19] Infliximab, adalimumab, and certolizumab pegol *(Cimzia)* are FDA-approved for treatment of moderate to severe CD.[20] Biosimilars for infliximab *(Inflectra, Renflexis, Ixifi)* and adalimumab (*Cyltezo*; not yet marketed) have been approved by the FDA.[21] Measuring drug and antibody levels in patients taking these drugs can be helpful, particularly in those with treatment failure.[22]

Efficacy in Ulcerative Colitis – TNF inhibitors are also effective for treatment of UC. Infliximab, adalimumab, and golimumab have all been

Table 3. Some Drugs for Inflammatory Bowel Disease

Drug	Some Formulations
Oral Aminosalicylates (5-ASAs)[2]	
Mesalamine	
Apriso (Salix)	375 mg ER caps
Asacol HD (Allergan)	800 mg DR tabs
generic	
Delzicol[3] (Allergan)	400 mg DR caps
Lialda (Shire)	1.2 g DR tabs
generic	
Pentasa (Shire)	250, 500 mg ER caps
5-ASA prodrugs	
Balsalazide – generic	750 mg caps
Colazal (Salix)	
Giazo (Salix)	1.1 g tabs
Olsalazine – *Dipentum* (Meda)	250 mg caps
Sulfasalazine – generic	500 mg tabs
Azulfidine (Pfizer)	
delayed-release – generic	500 mg enteric-coated DR tabs
Azulfidine En-tabs (Pfizer)	
Rectal Aminosalicylates	
Mesalamine	
generic	4 g/60 mL enema
Rowasa (Meda)	
SF Rowasa (Meda)	
Canasa (Allergan)	1000 mg rectal suppository

ER = extended-release; DR = delayed-release
1. Approximate WAC for 30 days' treatment at the lowest maintenance dosage. Prices for *Asacol HD, Pentasa, Giazo*, prednisone, hydrocortisone, and cyclosporine are based on the lowest induction dosage. WAC = wholesaler acquisition cost or manufacturer's published price to wholesalers; WAC represents a published catalogue or list price and may not represent an actual transactional price. Source: AnalySource® Monthly. June 5, 2018. Reprinted with permission by First Databank, Inc. All rights reserved. ©2018. www.fdbhealth.com/policies/drug-pricing-policy.

Usual Adult Dosage	Cost[1]
Maintenance: 1.5 g PO once/d	$481.40
Induction: 1.6 g PO tid	1545.70
	1117.60
Induction: 800 mg PO tid	425.20
Maintenance: 1.6 g PO daily in divided doses	
Induction: 2.4-4.8 g PO once/d	561.60
Maintenance: 2.4 g PO once/d	485.30
Induction: 1 g PO qid	1457.40
Induction: 2.25 g PO tid	111.30
Maintenance: 3-6 g PO daily in divided doses	669.10
Induction: 3.3 g PO bid	949.50
Induction: 1.5-3 g PO daily in 2 divided doses	1626.50
Maintenance: 500 mg PO bid	
Induction: 1 g PO qid	26.50
Maintenance: 1 g PO bid	181.10
Induction: 3-4 g PO daily in divided doses	31.90
Maintenance: 2 g PO daily in divided doses	236.60
Induction: 4 g rectally once/d at bedtime	366.50[4]
Maintenance: 2-4 g rectally once/d at bedtime	1508.90[4]
	1497.20[4]
Induction and maintenance: 1000 mg rectally once/d	1061.00

2. Not FDA-approved for use in Crohn's disease.
3. *Delzicol* has replaced *Asacol* due to reproductive safety concerns associated with dibutyl phthalate, a plasticizer in the enteric coating of *Asacol*. *Delzicol* does not contain dibutyl phthalate.
4. Cost for 28 days' treatment.

Continued on next page

Table 3. Some Drugs for Inflammatory Bowel Disease (continued)	
Drug	**Some Formulations**
Oral Corticosteroids	
Prednisone – generic	1, 2.5, 5, 10, 20, 50 mg tabs; 5 mg/5 mL, 5 mg/1 mL oral solution
delayed-release *Rayos* (Horizon)	1, 2, 5 mg DR tabs[5]
Budesonide – generic *Entocort EC* (Perrigo)[6]	3 mg caps
extended-release *Uceris* (Salix)[2]	9 mg ER tabs
Rectal Corticosteroids	
Budesonide *Uceris* (Salix)[2]	2 mg/actuation rectal foam

Hydrocortisone[2] – generic
  Colocort (Perrigo)
  Cortenema (Ani)
	100 mg/60 mL enema

Cortifoam (Meda)	10% rectal foam
Immunosuppressants[9]	

Azathioprine – generic
  Azasan (Salix)
  Imuran (Sebela)
	50 mg tabs
	75, 100 mg tabs
	50 mg tabs

Mercaptopurine – generic *Purixan* (Nova)	50 mg tabs 20 mg/mL oral susp
Methotrexate[11] – generic *Otrexup* (Antares)	25 mg/mL vials 15 mg, 17.5 mg, 20 mg, 22.5 mg, 25 mg/0.4 mL autoinjector
Rasuvo (Medac)	15 mg/0.3mL, 25 mg/0.5 mL autoinjector[13]
Cyclosporine – generic *Sandimmune* (Novartis)	50 mg/mL ampule

ER = extended-release; DR = delayed-release
5. The delayed-release tablets release active drug about 4 hours after ingestion.
6. Not FDA-approved for use in ulcerative colitis.
7. FDA-approved for up to 3 months.
8. Cost of two 15-gram aerosol containers (each contains ~14 applications).
9. Not FDA-approved for inflammatory bowel disease.

Usual Adult Dosage	Cost[1]
Induction: 40-60 mg PO once/d	$18.30
Induction: 40-60 mg PO once/d	20,080.00
Induction: 9 mg PO once/d	572.50
Maintenance: 6 mg PO once/d[7]	1380.90
Induction: 9 mg PO once/d	1792.80
Induction: 2 mg rectally bid x 2 wks	
Maintenance: 2 mg rectally once/d x 4 wks	512.00[4]
Induction: 1 enema rectally nightly	194.40
	255.80
	365.90
Induction: 1 application rectally once/d or bid	796.40[8]
Maintenance: 2-2.5 mg/kg PO once/d	41.60[10]
	317.40[10]
	602.30[10]
Maintenance: 1-1.5 mg/kg PO once/d	135.50[10]
	1277.50[10]
Induction: 25 mg IM/SC[12] once/wk	3.40
Maintenance: 15-25 mg IM/SC[12] once/wk	649.80
	470.00
Induction: 2-4 mg/kg IV daily	164.20[10,14]
	230.40[10,14]

10. Cost based on a 75-kg patient.
11. Use of supplements containing folic acid (1-4 mg daily) or folinic acid (2.5-10 mg weekly 24 hours after the methotrexate dose) may decrease adverse effects.
12. *Otrexup* and *Rasuvo* are for subcutaneous injection only.
13. Also available in 7.5 mg/0.15 mL, 10 mg/0.2 mL, 12.5 mg/0.15 mL, 17.5 mg/0.35 mL, 20 mg/0.4 mL, and 22.5 mg/0.45 mL.
14. Cost for 7 days' treatment.

Continued on next page

Table 3. Some Drugs for Inflammatory Bowel Disease (continued)

Drug	Some Formulations
TNF Inhibitors	
Adalimumab[15] – *Humira* (Abbvie)	40 mg/0.8 mL prefilled syringe; 40 mg/0.8 mL single-use pen
Certolizumab pegol[6] – *Cimzia* (UCB)	200 mg vial (lyophilized powder); 200 mg/mL prefilled syringe
Golimumab[2] – *Simponi* (Janssen)	50 mg/0.5 mL, 100 mg/1 mL auto-injector; 50 mg/0.5 mL, 100 mg/1 mL prefilled syringe
Infliximab – *Remicade* (Janssen) biosimilar Infliximab-abda – *Renflexis* (Merck) Infliximab-dyyb – *Inflectra* (Pfizer) Infliximab-qbtx – *Ixifi* (Pfizer)	100 mg vial (lyophilized powder)
Integrin Receptor Antagonists	
Natalizumab[6,17] – *Tysabri* (Elan/Biogen)	300 mg/15 mL vial (lyophilized powder)
Vedolizumab – *Entyvio* (Takeda)	300 mg/20 mL vial (lyophilized powder)
Interleukin (IL)-12 and -23 Antagonist	
Ustekinumab[2] – *Stelara* (Janssen)	130 mg/26 mL vial; 45 mg/0.5 mL vial; 45 mg/0.5 mL, 90 mg/1 mL prefilled syringes
Janus Kinase (JAK) Inhibitor	
Tofacitinib[2] – *Xeljanz* (Pfizer)	5, 10 mg tabs

N.A. = Not yet available
15. A biosimilar (adalimumab-adbm; *Cyltezo*) has been approved by the FDA, but is not yet marketed.
16. Cost for 8 weeks' treatment at the lowest maintenance dosage.
17. Providers must be registered with the *CD TOUCH* program to prescribe and dispense *Tysabri* for Crohn's disease.

Usual Adult Dosage	Cost[1]
Induction: 160 mg SC at wk 0, then 80 mg at wk 2 Maintenance: 40 mg SC every other wk starting at wk 4	$9744.00[16]
Induction: 400 mg SC at wks 0, 2, and 4 Maintenance: 400 mg SC q4 wks	8088.60[16]
Induction: 200 mg SC at wk 0, then 100 mg SC at wk 2 Maintenance: 100 mg SC q4 wks	10,395.50[16]
Induction: 5 mg/kg IV at wks 0, 2, and 6 Maintenance: 5-10 mg/kg IV q8 wks	4671.30[10,16]
	3013.60[10,16]
	3785.10[10,16]
	N.A.
Induction: 300 mg IV at wk 0 Maintenance: 300 mg IV q4 wks	12,360.00[16]
Induction: 300 mg IV at wks 0, 2, and 6 Maintenance: 300 mg IV q8 wks	5863.10[16]
Induction: 260, 390, or 520 mg[18] IV at wk 0 Maintenance: 90 mg SC q8 wks	20,584.30[16]
Induction: 10 mg PO bid for at least 8 wks[19] Maintenance: 5 or 10 mg PO bid[19,20]	8191.30[16]

18. 260 mg for patients <55 kg, 390 mg for those >55-85 kg, and 520 mg for patients >85 kg.
19. Dose reductions are needed for patients with moderate to severe renal impairment, moderate hepatic impairment, lymphopenia, neutropenia or anemia, and for those taking CYP2C19 and/or CYP3A4 inhibitors.
20. Discontinue if response is inadequate after 16 weeks of treatment with 10 mg twice daily.

shown to be significantly more effective than placebo in inducing and maintaining remission in patients with moderate to severe UC.[23] In a meta-analysis of clinical trials of biologic agents including infliximab, adalimumab, golimumab, and the integrin receptor antagonist vedolizumab *(Entyvio)*, there was no conclusive evidence that any one of these was more effective than any other in maintaining clinical remission in moderate to severe UC.[24]

Efficacy in Crohn's Disease – Infliximab has been effective for the treatment of moderate to severe CD that has not responded to other drugs, including systemic corticosteroids. It has been more effective than placebo in inducing and maintaining clinical and endoscopic remission and in producing closure of fistulas. Infliximab has also been shown to reduce CD recurrence after ileocolonic resection.[25]

Adalimumab and certolizumab pegol are also effective for induction and maintenance of remission in moderate to severe CD, but data comparing them to infliximab, or to each other, are lacking.[26-28]

Patients with primary nonresponse to one TNF inhibitor are unlikely to respond to another. In general, patients who are intolerant or have lost response to one TNF inhibitor, usually due to development of anti-drug antibodies, can be switched to another TNF inhibitor,[29,30] but the rate of response to a second TNF inhibitor is usually lower than the rate of response to the first. Use of an immunomodulator with a TNF inhibitor can reduce the formation of anti-drug antibodies.

In patients with CD in remission on infliximab, elective switching to adalimumab was associated with loss of efficacy.[31]

With Thiopurines – Use of a TNF inhibitor in combination with azathioprine or 6-MP may be more effective than use of either drug alone for treatment of UC and CD.[11,12]

Adverse Effects – Patients treated with TNF inhibitors are at increased risk for serious infections, including reactivated and disseminated tuberculosis, invasive or disseminated fungal infection, and other opportunistic infections, such as those caused by *Legionella* and *Listeria*. Tuberculin skin testing and chest radiography are recommended before starting treatment and periodically during therapy. Inhibition of TNF may result in reactivation of hepatitis B virus in patients who are chronic carriers; serologic testing for active hepatitis B infection is recommended before treatment. Anti-TNF therapies have also been associated with injection and infusion reactions and with new-onset psoriasis, hematologic cytopenias, non-ischemic congestive heart failure, demyelinating disorders, and induction of a lupus-like syndrome.

An increased risk of cancer, including lymphoma, melanoma, and non-melanoma skin cancers, has been reported with use of TNF inhibitors, but a causal relationship has not been established.[32] Long-term studies have not found an increased risk of malignancy in patients with IBD treated with anti-TNF therapy.[33-35]

Drug Interactions – Concomitant administration of a TNF inhibitor with another biologic agent may increase the risk of serious infections and neutropenia. Patients being treated with TNF inhibitors should not receive live vaccines.

INTERLEUKIN (IL)-12 AND -23 ANTAGONIST — Ustekinumab *(Stelara)* is an anti-p40 antibody that blocks IL-12 and -23. It is FDA-approved for treatment of patients with moderately to severely active CD after failure with corticosteroids, thiopurines, methotrexate, or TNF inhibitors.[36]

Efficacy – In clinical trials, ustekinumab induced a clinical response at week 6 in 34% and clinical remission at week 8 in 21% of patients with moderate to severe CD who were intolerant or had not responded to anti-TNF therapy, and in 56% and 40%, respectively, of patients who were intolerant or had not responded to immunosuppressants or corticosteroids.[37] Clinical remission was achieved in 53% of responders who continued ustekinumab for 44 weeks. In a long-term extension trial, the rates of CD-related hospitalization, surgery, and use of alternative biologic therapy at 96 weeks were significantly lower in patients who received ustekinumab every 8 weeks than in those who received placebo.[38]

Adverse Effects – The most common adverse effects of ustekinumab in clinical trials for CD were vomiting with induction treatment and nasopharyngitis, injection-site erythema, vulvovaginal candidiasis, bronchitis, pruritus, urinary tract infection, and sinusitis with maintenance treatment. Noninfectious interstitial pneumonia, eosinophilic pneumonia, and cryptogenic organizing pneumonia have been reported following one to three doses of the drug; some patients developed respiratory failure or required prolonged hospitalization. Ustekinumab has been associated with serious infections (including tuberculosis), malignancies, hypersensitivity reactions, and reversible posterior leukoencephalopathy syndrome. Screening for tuberculosis is recommended before starting treatment. Autoantibodies have developed; whether they reduce treatment response remains to be determined.

Drug Interactions – Administration of live vaccines should be avoided during treatment with ustekinumab. Proinflammatory cytokines can alter the formation of CYP isozymes; starting treatment with ustekinumab may normalize CYP isozyme formation and could alter serum concentrations of drugs that are CYP substrates.

INTEGRIN RECEPTOR ANTAGONISTS — Natalizumab *(Tysabri)* is FDA-approved for induction and maintenance treatment of moderate to severe CD. Vedolizumab *(Entyvio)* is FDA-approved for use in patients with CD or UC when corticosteroids, immunosuppressants, or TNF inhibitors have been ineffective or intolerable.[39] Vedolizumab is a humanized monoclonal antibody that binds to α4ß7 integrin. Blocking the α4ß7 integrin inhibits leukocyte migration into the GI tract, but not into the central nervous system, thereby decreasing the risk of progressive multifocal leukoencephalopathy (PML), which has occurred with natalizumab.

Table 4. Safety of Drugs for IBD in Pregnancy

Drug	Risk in Pregnancy[1]
Aminosalicylates	Most formulations generally considered safe Sulfasalazine can cause reversible oligospermia; stop 4 months before conception Pregnant women taking sulfasalazine may need higher doses of folic acid Fetal developmental toxicity has occurred when pregnant rats were given high doses
Corticosteroids	Data are conflicting, but experts suggest the risks associated with disease outweigh the low risk of adverse pregnancy outcomes Budesonide may result in lower fetal exposure than systemic corticosteroids
Thiopurines	Adverse pregnancy outcomes have been reported, but recent data suggests that use of azathioprine or mercaptopurine is not associated with adverse birth outcomes[2,3]
Methotrexate	Contraindicated; avoid pregnancy if either partner is taking methotrexate
Cyclosporine	Embryofetal toxicity in animals at high doses Congenital malformations not found in pregnant women treated with the drug after an organ transplant
TNF Inhibitors	Not associated with adverse pregnancy outcomes Placental transfer of anti-TNF antibodies higher in late second and third trimesters, especially with infliximab, adalimumab, and golimumab In women at low risk for relapse, consider stopping the TNF inhibitor at 22 weeks' gestation
Ustekinumab	No adequate studies in pregnant women No teratogenic effects in monkeys
Integrin Receptor Antagonists	No adequate studies in pregnant women with vedolizumab or natalizumab No fetal harm in animal studies with vedolizumab Fetal immunologic and hematologic adverse effects and fetal mortality in animal studies with natalizumab
Tofacitinib	No adequate studies in pregnant women Teratogenic effects and fetal deaths in animal studies

1. GC Nguyen et al. Gastroenterology 2016; 150:734.
2. MJ Casanova et al. Am J Gastroenterol 2013; 108:433.
3. J Coelho et al. Gut 2011; 60:198.

Efficacy in Crohn's Disease – **Natalizumab** has been modestly effective in some studies as an induction agent in patients with moderate to severe CD with active inflammation. It appears to be more effective at maintaining response and remission, with significant steroid-sparing effects.[40] Its use is limited to patients with negative JC virus testing because of the risk of PML.

In clinical trials in patients with moderate to severe CD who could not tolerate or had an inadequate response to prior treatment, induction treatment with **vedolizumab** resulted in a clinical response in 31% and clinical remission in 15% of patients at week 6; 39% of responders were in remission at 52 weeks.[41]

Efficacy in Ulcerative Colitis – Clinical response at week 6 was achieved in 47% of patients with UC who received induction treatment with vedolizumab, and 42% of patients treated with the drug were in clinical remission at 52 weeks.[42]

A meta-analysis found that after 12 months of treatment with vedolizumab, 46% of patients with UC and 30% with CD were in remission.[43]

Adverse Effects – Use of natalizumab has been limited by the rare occurence of PML and severe hepatic toxicity; JC virus antibody testing should be performed every 6 months during treatment with the drug. No cases of PML have been reported with vedolizumab to date.

Hypersensitivity reactions including anaphylaxis have been reported with both drugs. Severe infections including tuberculosis and meningitis have also occurred. Increased transaminase and bilirubin levels have been reported.

Drug Interactions – Other biologic agents or immunomodulators may increase the risk of infectious complications with natalizumab or vedolizumab and should not be used concomitantly.

JANUS KINASE (JAK) INHIBITOR — The oral JAK inhibitor tofacitinib *(Xeljanz)* was recently approved by the FDA for treatment of moderate to severe UC in adults.

Efficacy – In two unpublished, double-blind trials (summarized in the package insert) in patients with moderate to severe UC who were intolerant or had failed treatment with systemic corticosteroids, azathioprine, 6-MP, or a TNF inhibitor, induction treatment with tofacitinib resulted in remission at 8 weeks in 18% of patients in study 1 and in 17% of patients in study 2. In a maintenance trial in patients who completed tofacitinib induction treatment and achieved a clinical response, 34% of patients taking tofacitinib 5 mg twice daily and 41% of patients taking 10 mg twice daily were in remission at 52 weeks.

Adverse Effects – Common adverse effects of tofacitinib in clinical trials for UC included nasopharyngitis, upper respiratory tract infection, increased blood creatine phosphokinase, elevated cholesterol levels, rash, headache, diarrhea, and herpes zoster. Severe, sometimes fatal, infections have occurred. Tuberculosis and other opportunistic infections have been reported; patients should be tested for latent or active tuberculosis before starting tofacitinib. Lymphocytopenia, neutropenia, and low hemoglobin levels can occur in patients taking tofacitinib. Lymphocytes should be monitored at baseline and then every 3 months, and neutrophil and hemoglobin levels should be monitored at baseline, after 4-8 weeks of treatment, and then every 3 months.

In a long-term safety study in patients with UC, malignancies were reported more often in patients taking tofacitinib 10 mg than in those taking the 5-mg dose. GI perforation has been reported during clinical trials with tofacitinib for other indications.

Drug Interactions – Tofacitinib is metabolized by CYP3A4. Strong inhibitors of CYP3A4,[8] such as clarithromycin *(Biaxin, and others)*, can increase tofacitinib serum concentrations; the dosage of tofacitinib should be reduced in patients taking a strong CYP3A4 inhibitor concurrently. Drugs that are both moderate CYP3A4 and strong CYP2C19 inhibitors, such as fluconazole (*Diflucan*, and generics), also increase serum concentrations of tofacitinib; the dosage of tofacitinib should be reduced if these drugs are taken concurrently. Potent inducers of CYP3A4, such as rifampin (*Rifadin*, and generics), decrease tofacitinib levels and concomitant use should be avoided. Tofacitinib should not be used with other biologic agents or potent immunosuppressant drugs such as azathioprine. Live vaccines should not be given to patients taking tofacitinib; vaccinations should be updated before starting treatment.

ANTIBIOTICS AND PROBIOTICS — Many experts believe that alterations in the balance of enteric bacteria (dysbiosis) play a role in the development of IBD, but evidence that **antibiotics** are effective in treating CD or UC is limited, and they may make dysbiosis worse.[44] Metronidazole (*Flagyl*, and generics) and ciprofloxacin (*Cipro*, and generics) are often used, sometimes together, to treat CD microperforations and fistulas. They have also been used following resections to prevent recurrence of CD.[45,46] Antibiotics are not recommended for the treatment of luminal CD. Antibiotic treatment is recommended for patients with UC who develop pouchitis following colectomy and ileoanal pouch formation.[47]

Probiotics, such as *VSL #3*, may maintain remission in UC patients with pouchitis after ileoanal anastomosis for severe disease.[48,49] They have not been found to be effective for management of CD.

1. B Bressler et al. Clinical practice guidelines for the medical management of nonhospitalized ulcerative colitis: the Toronto consensus. Gastroenterol 2015; 148:1035.
2. A Kornbluth et al. Ulcerative colitis practice guidelines in adults: American College of Gastroenterology, Practice Parameters Committee. Am J Gastroenterol 2010; 105:501.
3. GR Lichtenstein et al. ACG clinical guideline: management of Crohn's disease in adults. Am J Gastroenterol 2018; 113:481.
4. AC Ford et al. Efficacy of 5-aminosalicylates in ulcerative colitis: systematic review and meta-analysis. Am J Gastroenterol 2011; 106:601.

5. GT Ho et al. The efficacy of corticosteroid therapy in inflammatory bowel disease: analysis of a 5-year UK inception cohort. Aliment Pharmacol Ther 2006; 24:319.
6. Budesonide (Uceris) for ulcerative colitis. Med Lett Drugs Ther 2013; 55:23.
7. Budesonide rectal foam (Uceris) for ulcerative colitis. Med Lett Drugs Ther 2015; 57:154.
8. Inhibitors and inducers of CYP enzymes and P-glycoprotein. Med Lett Drugs Ther 2017 Sept 18 (epub). Available at: www.medicalletter.org/downloads/CYP_PGP_Tables.pdf. Accessed June 22, 2018.
9. A Timmer et al. Azathioprine and 6-mercaptopurine for maintenance of remission in ulcerative colitis. Cochrane Database Syst Rev 2012; 9:CD000478.
10. E Prefontaine et al. Azathioprine or 6-mercaptopurine for maintenance of remission in Crohn's disease. Cochrane Database Syst Rev 2009; 1:CD000067.
11. JF Colombel et al. Infliximab, azathioprine, or combination therapy for Crohn's disease. N Engl J Med 2010; 362:1383.
12. R Panaccione et al. Combination therapy with infliximab and azathioprine is superior to monotherapy with either agent in ulcerative colitis. Gastroenterology 2014; 146:392.
13. AM Abbas et al. Risk of melanoma and non-melanoma skin cancer in ulcerative colitis patients treated with thiopurines: a nationwide retrospective cohort. Am J Gastroenterol 2014; 109:1781.
14. M Lemaitre et al. Association between use of thiopurines or tumor necrosis factor antagonists alone or in combination and risk of lymphoma in patients with inflammatory bowel disease. JAMA 2017; 318:1679.
15. A Vasudevan et al. Low-dose thiopurine with allopurinol co-therapy overcomes thiopurine intolerance and allows thiopurine continuation in inflammatory bowel disease. Dig Liv Dis 2018 Feb 10 (epub).
16. JW McDonald et al. Methotrexate for induction of remission in refractory Crohn's disease. Cochrane Database Syst Rev 2014; 8:CD003459.
17. BG Feagan et al. Methotrexate in combination with infliximab is no more effective than infliximab alone in patients with Crohn's disease. Gastroenterology 2014; 146:681.
18. I Ordás et al. Long-term efficacy and safety of cyclosporine in a cohort of steroid-refractory acute severe ulcerative colitis patients from the ENEIDA Registry (1989-2013): a nationwide multicenter study. Am J Gastroenterol 2017; 112:1709.
19. Golimumab (Simponi) for ulcerative colitis. Med Lett Drugs Ther 2014; 56:25.
20. TNF inhibitors for Crohn's disease: when, which, and for how long. Med Lett Drugs Ther 2013; 55:102.
21. Inflectra – an infliximab biosimilar. Med Lett Drugs Ther 2017; 59:23.
22. JD Feuerstein et al. American Gastroenterological Association Institute guideline on therapeutic drug monitoring in inflammatory bowel disease. Gastroenterol 2017; 153:827.
23. WJ Sandborn et al. Subcutaneous golimumab induces clinical response and remission in patients with moderate-to-severe ulcerative colitis. Gastroenterology 2014; 146:85.
24. S Danese et al. Biological agents for moderately to severely active ulcerative colitis: a systematic review and network meta-analysis. Ann Intern Med 2014; 160:704.
25. M Regueiro et al. Postoperative therapy with infliximab prevents long-term Crohn's disease recurrence. Clin Gastroenterol Hepatol 2014; 12:1494.
26. JF Colombel et al. Adalimumab for maintenance of clinical response and remission in patients with Crohn's disease: the CHARM trial. Gastroenterology 2007; 132:52.

27. WJ Sandborn et al. Adalimumab induction therapy for Crohn disease previously treated with infliximab: a randomized trial. Ann Intern Med 2007; 146:829.
28. S Schreiber et al. Maintenance therapy with certolizumab pegol for Crohn's disease. N Engl J Med 2007; 357:239.
29. R Panaccione et al. Clinical benefit of long-term adalimumab treatment in patients with Crohn's disease following loss of response or intolerance to infliximab: 96-week efficacy data from GAIN/ADHERE trials. J Crohns Colitis 2018 April 25 (epub).
30. WJ Sandborn et al. Certolizumab pegol in patients with moderate to severe Crohn's disease and secondary failure to infliximab. Clin Gastroenterol Hepatol 2010; 8:688.
31. G Van Assche et al. Switch to adalimumab in patients with Crohn's disease controlled by maintenance infliximab: prospective randomised SWITCH trial. Gut 2012; 61:229.
32. X Mariette et al. Malignancies associated with tumour necrosis factor inhibitors in registries and prospective observational studies: a systematic review and meta-analysis. Ann Rheum Dis 2011; 70:1895.
33. N Nyboe Andersen et al. Association between tumor necrosis factor-α antagonists and risk of cancer in patients with inflammatory bowel disease. JAMA 2014; 311:2406.
34. GR Lichtenstein et al. Infliximab for Crohn's disease: more than 13 years of real-world experience. Inflamm Bowel Dis 2018; 24:490.
35. G D'Haens et al. Lymphoma risk and overall safety profile of adalimumab in patients with Crohn's disease with up to 6 years of follow-up in the Pyramid Registry. Am J Gastroenterol 2018 June 5 (epub).
36. Ustekinumab (Stelara) for Crohn's disease. Med Lett Drugs Ther 2017; 59:5.
37. B Feagan et al. Ustekinumab as induction and maintenance therapy for Crohn's disease. N Engl J Med 2016; 375:1946.
38. WJ Sandborn et al. Reduced rates of Crohn's-related surgeries, hospitalizations and alternate biologic initiation with uskekinumab in the IM-UNITI study through 2 years. Gastroenterology 2018; 154:S377. Abstract Sa1743.
39. Vedolizumab (Entyvio) for inflammatory bowel disease. Med Lett Drugs Ther 2014; 56:86.
40. Natalizumab (Tysabri) for Crohn's disease. Med Lett Drugs Ther 2008; 50:34.
41. WJ Sandborn et al. Vedolizumab as induction and maintenance therapy for Crohn's disease. N Engl J Med 2013; 369:711.
42. BG Feagan et al. Vedolizumab as induction and maintenance therapy for ulcerative colitis. N Engl J Med 2013; 369:699.
43. S Schreiber et al. Systematic review with meta-analysis: real-world effectiveness and safety of vedolizumab in patients with inflammatory bowel disease. J Gastroenterol 2018 June 4 (epub).
44. D Gevers et al. The treatment-naive microbiome in new-onset Crohn's disease. Cell Host Microbe 2014; 15:382.
45. HH Herfarth et al. Ciprofloxacin for the prevention of postoperative recurrence in patients with Crohn's disease: a randomized, double-blind, placebo-controlled pilot study. Inflamm Bowel Dis 2013; 19:1073.
46. M Mañosa et al. Addition of metronidazole to azathioprine for the prevention of postoperative recurrence of Crohn's disease: a randomized, double-blind, placebo-controlled trial. Inflamm Bowel Dis 2013; 19:1889.

47. RL Dalal et al. Management of pouchitis and other common complications of the pouch. Inflamm Bowel Dis 2018; 24:989.
48. Y Derwa et al. Systematic review with meta-analysis: the efficacy of probiotics in inflammatory bowel disease. Aliment Pharmacol Ther 2017; 46:389.
49. S Singh et al. Treatment and prevention of pouchitis after ileal pouch-anal anastomosis for chronic ulcerative colitis. Cochrane Database Syst Rev 2015; 11:CD001176.

DRUGS FOR
Chronic Insomnia

Original publication date – December 2018

Cognitive behavioral therapy for insomnia (CBT-I) is recommended for initial treatment of chronic insomnia. Pharmacologic treatment should be used in addition to CBT-I when CBT-I alone is not effective.[1-3]

BENZODIAZEPINE RECEPTOR AGONISTS — Eszopiclone (*Lunesta*, and generics), zaleplon (*Sonata,* and generics), and zolpidem (*Ambien*, and others) decrease sleep latency and are FDA-approved for short-term treatment of sleep-onset insomnia. Eszopiclone and the extended-release formulation of zolpidem (*Ambien CR*, and generics) are also approved for sleep-maintenance insomnia. The low-dose sublingual formulation of zolpidem (*Intermezzo*, and generics) is the only hypnotic FDA-approved for treatment of insomnia following middle-of-the-night awakening,[4] but zaleplon, which has a similar duration of action, is often used off-label for this purpose.

Adverse Effects – Headache and dizziness are common adverse effects of benzodiazepine receptor agonists. Eszopiclone can leave an unpleasant aftertaste.

In 2013, the FDA required manufacturers of zolpidem-containing products to lower the recommended dose for women and to recommend consideration of a lower dose for men because of concerns about impaired next-day performance, including driving.[5,6] No change was required in

---

Recommendations for Treatment of Chronic Insomnia

▸ Cognitive behavioral therapy for insomnia (CBT-I) is recommended for first-line treatment of chronic insomnia.

▸ Pharmacologic treatment can be used in addition to CBT-I in patients who continue to have insomnia despite CBT-I.

▸ A short-acting benzodiazepine receptor agonist such as zaleplon or zolpidem is a reasonable choice for treatment of sleep-onset insomnia. Ramelteon is an alternative, but its efficacy appears to be limited.

▸ An intermediate- or a long-acting drug, such as eszopiclone, extended-release zolpidem, low-dose doxepin, or suvorexant, can be used for treatment of sleep-maintenance insomnia, but impairment of next-day performance can occur.

▸ Zaleplon and the low-dose sublingual formulation of zolpidem *(Intermezzo)* can be used for insomnia following middle-of-the-night awakening.

▸ Tolerance and dependence occur with prolonged use of benozdiazepines. Their use for treatment of chronic insomnia should be discouraged, particularly in older patients and those with sleep apnea or a history of substance abuse.

▸ There is little evidence to support the use of antidepressants, such as trazodone, for treatment of insomnia in patients without comorbid depression.

▸ Second-generation antipsychotics have many adverse effects and are not recommended for treatment of chronic insomnia in patients without a comorbid psychiatric illness.

▸ Antihistamines can impair next-day performance and are not recommended for treatment of chronic insomnia.

▸ Over-the-counter dietary supplements, such as melatonin, and herbal products have been used as sleep aids, but the purity of these products and optimal dosages are unclear.

---

the dose of *Intermezzo* because it was approved at a low dose. The FDA has also recommended reducing the starting dose of eszopiclone to 1 mg for both men and women because an evening dose of 3 mg can impair driving skills, memory, and coordination for more than 11 hours.[7]

Complex sleep-related behaviors without conscious awareness, such as sleep-walking, sleep-eating, and sleep-driving, have occurred with use of benzodiazepine receptor agonists[8,9]; risk factors include use of the drug in high doses, with other sedating drugs, or while still active.[10] Use of these drugs in elderly patients has been associated with adverse cognitive effects and an increased risk of falls. Observational cohort studies have found that use of hypnotics, particularly zolpidem, has been associated with an increased risk of cancer and death[11,12]; a causal relationship has not been established. Benzodiazepine receptor agonists are classified as schedule IV controlled substances; withdrawal, dependence, and abuse can occur.

Drug Interactions – Eszopiclone, zolpidem, and (to a lesser extent) zaleplon are metabolized by CYP3A4. Concurrent administration of a strong CYP3A4 inhibitor, such as clarithromycin (*Biaxin*, and others), could increase their serum concentrations and the risk of adverse effects. Concurrent use of a strong CYP3A4 inducer, such as rifampin (*Rifadin*, and others), could decrease their effectiveness and is not recommended.[13] Concurrent use of a benzodiazepine receptor agonist and alcohol or other CNS depressants increases the risk of CNS depression.

Pregnancy and Lactation – Preterm birth and low birth weights have been reported in the offspring of women who took a benzodiazepine receptor agonist during pregnancy.[14] Use of zolpidem in the third trimester has resulted in respiratory depression and sedation in neonates.

Zaleplon and zolpidem have been detected in human breast milk, and excess sedation has been reported in breastfed infants of mothers who took zolpidem.

BENZODIAZEPINES — Benzodiazepines differ in their onset and durations of action. They all decrease sleep latency and prolong the first two stages of sleep. Tolerance to the sedative effects of benzodiazepines develops rapidly; these drugs are not recommended for long-term use.

Adverse Effects – Benzodiazepines can impair next-day performance, including driving.[15] Complex sleep-related behaviors without conscious awareness and anterograde amnesia can occur, particularly with triazolam (*Halcion*, and generics). Aggressive behavior has been reported.[16] In elderly patients, benzodiazepines can cause weakness and impair coordination, and their use as hypnotics has been associated with

Table 1. Some Oral Hypnotics for Chronic Insomnia

Drug	Oral Formulations	Onset of Action
Benzodiazepine Receptor Agonists[4]		
Eszopiclone – generic Lunesta (Sunovion)	1, 2, 3 mg tabs	<30 min[5]
Zaleplon – generic Sonata (Pfizer)	5, 10 mg caps	<30 min
Zolpidem – immediate-release – generic Ambien (Sanofi)	5, 10 mg tabs	<30 min[5]
extended-release – generic Ambien CR	6.25, 12.5 mg ER tabs	<30 min[5]
spray – Zolpimist (Aytu Bioscience)	5 mg/spray	20 min[5]
sublingual – Edluar (Meda)	5, 10 mg SL tabs	<30 min[5]
Intermezzo (Purdue) generic	1.75, 3.5 mg SL tabs	20 min[5]
Benzodiazepines[9]		
Estazolam – generic	1, 2 mg tabs	15-60 min
Flurazepam – generic	15, 30 mg caps	10-30 min
Lorazepam[10] – generic Ativan (Valeant)	0.5, 1, 2 mg tabs	30-60 min
Quazepam – generic Doral (Galt)	15 mg tabs	30 min
Temazepam – generic Restoril (Mallinckrodt)	7.5, 15, 22.5, 30 mg caps	30-60 min
Triazolam – generic Halcion (Pfizer)	0.125, 0.25 mg tabs 0.25 mg tabs	15-30 min

ER = extended-release; SL = sublingual
1. Treatment should be started with the lowest dose, especially in patients who have a low body weight, are debilitated, or are receiving opioids or other CNS or cardiorespiratory depressants.
2. Dosage adjustment may be required for renal or hepatic impairment.
3. Approximate WAC for 30 days' treatment at the lowest usual adult hypnotic dosage. WAC = wholesaler acquisition cost or manufacturer's published price to wholesalers; WAC represents a published catalogue or list price and may not represent an actual transactional price. Source: AnalySource® Monthly. December 5, 2018. Reprinted with permission by First Databank, Inc. All rights reserved. ©2018. www.fdbhealth.com/policies/drug-pricing-policy.
4. Eszopiclone and extended-release zolpidem are FDA-approved for treatment of sleep-onset and sleep-maintenance insomnia. Intermezzo is only approved for insomnia following middle-of-the-night awakening. Zaleplon and the immediate-release, sublingual (Edluar), and spray formulations of zolpidem are FDA-approved for treatment of sleep-onset insomnia.

Duration	Usual Adult Hypnotic Dose[1,2]	Dose in Elderly[2]	Cost[3]
intermediate	1-3 mg	1-2 mg	$19.20 470.40
ultra-short	10-20 mg[6]	5 mg[6]	9.50 322.90
short	men: 5-10 mg women: 5 mg	5 mg	2.40 504.90
intermediate	men: 6.25-12.5 mg women: 6.25 mg	6.25 mg	22.50 504.90
short	men: 5-10 mg[7] women: 5 mg[7]	5 mg[7]	659.00[8]
short	men: 5-10 mg women: 5 mg	5 mg	356.20
ultra-short	men: 3.5 mg[7] women: 1.75 mg[7]	1.75 mg[7]	372.30 237.10
intermediate	1-2 mg	0.5-1 mg	33.50
long	15-30 mg	15 mg	14.90
intermediate	0.5-2 mg	0.5-1 mg	1.80 699.30
long	7.5-15 mg	7.5 mg	281.30[11] 705.00[11]
intermediate	7.5-30 mg	7.5-15 mg	121.00 924.10
short	0.125-0.25 mg	0.125-0.25 mg	87.90 83.90[12]

5. Onset may be slower if taken with or immediately after a meal.
6. Should not be taken with or immediately after a high-fat meal.
7. Should only be taken if ≥4 hours remain before waking.
8. Cost of a 7.7-mL bottle that contains 60 5-mg actuations after 5 initial priming actuations.
9. Estazolam, flurazepam, quazepam, and temazepam are FDA-approved for treatment of sleep-onset and sleep-maintenance insomnia. Triazolam is only approved for treatment of sleep-onset insomnia. Quazepam and its metabolites have long half-lives, which can lead to toxicity and next-day impairment; it is generally not recommended for treatment of chronic insomnia.
10. Lorazepam is not FDA-approved for treatment of insomnia.
11. Cost of 15 15-mg tablets.
12. Cost of 15 0.25-mg tablets.

Continued on next page

Table 1. Some Oral Hypnotics for Chronic Insomnia (continued)		
Drug	Oral Formulations	Onset of Action
Melatonin Receptor Agonist[13]		
Ramelteon – *Rozerem* (Takeda)	8 mg tabs	15-30 min
Tricyclic Antidepressant[14]		
Doxepin – *Silenor* (Pernix)	3, 6 mg tabs	30 min
Orexin Receptor Antagonist[16]		
Suvorexant – *Belsomra* (Merck)	5, 10, 15, 20 mg tabs	30 min[5]
13. Ramelteon is FDA-approved for treatment of sleep-onset insomnia. 14. Doxepin is FDA-approved for treatment of sleep-maintenance insomnia.		

an increased incidence of falls and hip fractures. Benzodiazepines are classified as schedule IV controlled substances. Dependence, tolerance, abuse, and rebound insomnia can occur with their use. Withdrawal, which may be life-threatening, can occur with rapid dosage reductions or abrupt discontinuation.

Drug Interactions – All benzodiazepines, except lorazepam, oxazepam, and temazepam, are metabolized to some extent by CYP3A4. Inhibitors of CYP3A4, such as clarithromycin, can increase benzodiazepine serum concentrations and the risk of toxicity, and inducers, such as rifampin, can decrease their serum concentrations and possibly their effectiveness.[13] Alcohol and other CNS depressants increase the risk of benzodiazepine-induced CNS depression. Concurrent use of an opioid and a benzodiazepine has been associated with a significant increase in the risk of overdose compared to use of an opioid alone.[17]

Pregnancy and Lactation – Benzodiazepines increase the risk of fetal malformations; they should not be taken during pregnancy.

The American College of Obstetricians and Gynecologists (ACOG) considers benzodiazepines moderately safe for use during breastfeeding.[18]

Duration	Usual Adult Hypnotic Dose[1,2]	Dose in Elderly[2]	Cost[3]
short	8 mg[6]	8 mg[6]	$377.70
long	3-6 mg[15]	3 mg[15]	428.30
intermediate	10-20 mg	10-20 mg	331.50

15. Should not be taken within 3 hours of a meal.
16. Suvorexant is FDA-approved for treatment of sleep-onset and sleep-maintenance insomnia.

MELATONIN RECEPTOR AGONIST — The melatonin receptor agonist ramelteon *(Rozerem)* is FDA-approved for treatment of sleep-onset insomnia, but its efficacy for this indication is modest at best.[19] It does not appear to be effective for treatment of sleep-maintenance insomnia.

Adverse Effects – Common adverse effects of ramelteon include somnolence, dizziness, fatigue, and nausea. Hallucinations, agitation, mania, and complex sleep-related behaviors without conscious awareness have been reported. Increased serum prolactin and decreased serum testosterone concentrations can occur. Ramelteon is not classified as a controlled substance.

Pregnancy and Lactation – There are no adequate studies on the use of ramelteon in pregnant women. Developmental toxicity and teratogenic effects have occurred in the offspring of pregnant rats given ramelteon at doses much higher than the recommended human dose.

There are no data on the presence of ramelteon in human breast milk or on its effects on the breastfed infant or milk production. Ramelteon is excreted in the milk of lactating rats.

Drug Interactions – Ramelteon is metabolized by CYP1A2 and to a lesser extent by CYP2C and 3A4 isozymes. Administration of the selective serotonin reuptake inhibitor (SSRI) fluvoxamine (*Luvox*, and others), which is a strong CYP1A2 inhibitor, markedly increases ramelteon serum concentrations; concurrent use of the two drugs is contraindicated. Other CYP1A2 inhibitors, such as ciprofloxacin (*Cipro*, and others), could have a similar effect. Drugs that inhibit CYP3A4 or 2C9 could also increase ramelteon serum concentrations and the risk of toxicity.[13] Rifampin, a potent inducer of various CYP isozymes, decreases ramelteon serum concentrations by 80%. Concurrent use of ramelteon and alcohol or other CNS depressants increases the risk of CNS depression.

LOW-DOSE DOXEPIN — The tricyclic antidepressant doxepin *(Silenor)* is FDA-approved for treatment of sleep-maintenance insomnia. Its affinity for H_1-histamine receptors is thought to be largely responsible for its sedating effect. In doses much lower than those used to treat depression (3-6 mg vs 150-300 mg), it is claimed to have a hypnotic effect without causing anticholinergic and other typical tricyclic adverse effects. Clinical studies have demonstrated efficacy in both healthy volunteers (51 minutes more total sleep time) and in elderly patients with chronic insomnia.[20]

Adverse Effects – Residual next-day somnolence has been reported with the 6-mg dose. Doxepin is not classified as a controlled substance.

Drug Interactions – Coadministration with cimetidine (*Tagamet*, and others), an inhibitor of CYP2C19, 2D6, and 1A2, can double doxepin serum concentrations; a maximum doxepin dose of 3 mg is recommended for patients also taking cimetidine. Doxepin is contraindicated for use with a monoamine oxidase inhibitor (MAOI) or within two weeks of stopping one. Concurrent use of alcohol or other CNS depressants can increase the risk of CNS depression.

Pregnancy and Lactation – There are no adequate studies on the use of low-dose doxepin in pregnant women. Administration of doxepin ≥6 mg/day to pregnant rats resulted in adverse effects on fetal development.

Doxepin is excreted in human breast milk. Apnea and drowsiness were reported in an infant whose mother was taking doxepin in doses used to treat depression. The effect of doxepin on milk production is unknown.

OREXIN RECEPTOR ANTAGONIST — Suvorexant *(Belsomra)*, the orexin receptor antagonist, is FDA-approved for treatment of both sleep-onset and sleep-maintenance insomnia. Signaling of orexin neuropeptides sustains wakefulness.[21] Suvorexant promotes sleep by blocking orexin neuropeptides from binding to their receptors. Clinical trials have shown that patients treated with the drug fall asleep 5-10 minutes sooner and stay asleep 15-25 minutes longer than those taking placebo.[22] Loss of orexin signaling has been associated with narcolepsy; suvorexant is contraindicated for use in patients with narcolepsy.

Adverse Effects – The most common adverse effects of suvorexant are somnolence, fatigue, and abnormal dreams.[23] Suvorexant has a long half-life and can impair next-day performance, including driving. Complex sleep-related behaviors and cataplexy-like symptoms, such as leg weakness, have been reported. Suvorexant should be administered with caution to patients with compromised respiratory function; it appears to be safe for use in patients with mild to moderate COPD.[24] Suvorexant is classified as a schedule IV controlled substance.

Drug Interactions – Suvorexant is a CYP3A4 substrate and should not be administered with strong CYP3A4 inhibitors, such as clarithromycin. In patients taking moderate CYP3A4 inhibitors, such as fluconazole *(Diflucan*, and generics), verapamil *(Calan*, and others), or grapefruit juice, the recommended dose of suvorexant is 5 mg, which can be increased to 10 mg if needed. The efficacy of suvorexant may be reduced in patients concomitantly taking a strong CYP3A4 inducer, such as carbamazepine *(Tegretol*, and others).[13] Suvorexant is a P-glycoprotein (P-gp) inhibitor; it can increase digoxin serum concentrations if taken concomitantly. Concurrent use of suvorexant and alcohol or other CNS depressants increases the risk of CNS depression.

Pregnancy and Lactation – There are no adequate studies on the use of suvorexant in pregnant women. Administration of higher-than-recommended doses of the drug to pregnant rats has resulted in reduced fetal weight in their offspring.

There are no data on the presence of suvorexant in human breast milk or on its effects on the breastfed infant or milk production. Suvorexant has been detected in the milk of lactating rats at concentrations higher than those in plasma.

OTHER PRESCRIPTION DRUGS — Many drugs are used off-label for treatment of insomnia. The most common are **antidepressants** such as trazodone (*Desyrel,* and generics), mirtazapine (*Remeron,* and generics), and amitriptyline (*Elavil,* and generics). There is little evidence that these drugs are effective in treating insomnia not associated with depression.[25,26] Second-generation **antipsychotics**, such as quetiapine (*Seroquel*, and others), have also been used for treatment of insomnia, but their risks outweigh their benefits in patients without a comorbid psychiatric condition.[27,28] The **antiepileptic/neuropathic analgesics** gabapentin (*Neurontin*, and others) and pregabalin *(Lyrica)* have been shown to increase slow-wave sleep and sleep efficiency; they could be considered for treatment of patients with comorbid conditions such as restless legs syndrome or fibromyalgia.[29]

ANTIHISTAMINES — The first-generation antihistamines diphenhydramine (*Nytol*, *Benadryl*, *Unisom,* and others) and doxylamine (*Unisom Sleep Tabs*, and others) are marketed for over-the-counter sale as "sleep aids". These drugs are sedating, but there is little acceptable evidence that they improve the quality or duration of sleep. Tolerance to their sedative effects may develop rapidly. Antihistamines can cause next-day impairment of performance skills such as driving, and anticholinergic adverse effects, such as dry mouth and urinary retention, which may be particularly troublesome in elderly patients.[30] These drugs are sometimes used for treatment of insomnia during pregnancy.

ALCOHOL — Although widely used as a hypnotic, alcohol causes CNS depression initially followed by rebound excitation, which disrupts sleep. Self-medication with alcohol to relieve insomnia can lead to development of alcoholism.

MELATONIN — Taken 3-5 hours before the desired time of sleep onset, melatonin has been reported to be effective in some patients with sleep-onset insomnia. It does not appear to be effective when taken at bedtime. A sustained-release formulation of melatonin *(Circadin)* is available in Europe; one study found it to be more effective than placebo when taken 2 hours before bedtime in patients ≥65 years old.[31]

HERBAL PRODUCTS — **Valerian root** is claimed to be a mild hypnotic that may improve the quality of sleep, but some studies have found it ineffective.[32] There is no convincing evidence that any of the other "natural" remedies used for insomnia, such as **kava** or **lavender**, are effective or safe for this indication and the purity and optimal dosages of all these products are unknown.[33] No objective data have been published to date to support the subjective claim of sleep improvement attributed to **cannabis** or its various extracts.

1. A Qaseem et al. Management of chronic insomnia disorder in adults: a clinical practice guideline from the American College of Physicians. Ann Intern Med 2016; 165:125.
2. DJ Buysse et al. Clinical management of insomnia disorder. JAMA 2017; 318:1973.
3. MJ Sateia et al. Clinical practice guideline for the pharmacologic treatment of chronic insomnia in adults: an American Academy of Sleep Medicine Clinical Practice Guideline. J Clin Sleep Med 2017; 13:307.
4. Low-dose sublingual zolpidem (Intermezzo) for insomnia due to middle-of-the-night awakening. Med Lett Drugs Ther 2012; 54:25.
5. FDA requires lower dosing of zolpidem. Med Lett Drugs Ther 2013; 55:5.
6. FDA Drug Safety Communication: FDA approves new label changes and dosing for zolpidem products and a recommendation to avoid driving the day after using Ambien CR. Available at: www.fda.gov/Drugs/DrugSafety/ucm352085.htm. Accessed December 6, 2018.
7. In brief: lowering the dose of Lunesta. Med Lett Drugs Ther 2014; 56:48.
8. N Gunja. In the Zzz zone: the effects of Z-drugs on human performance and driving. J Med Toxicol 2013; 9:163.
9. N Gunja. The clinical and forensic toxicology of Z-drugs. J Med Toxicol 2013; 9:155.

10. JS Poceta. Zolpidem ingestion, automatisms, and sleep driving: a clinical and legal case series. J Clin Sleep Med 2011; 7:632.

11. DF Kripke et al. Hypnotics' association with mortality or cancer: a matched cohort study. BMJ Open 2012; 2:e000850.

12. SC Lin et al. Zolpidem increased cancer risk in patients with sleep disorder: a 3-year follow-up study. J Med Sci 2016; 36:68.

13. Inhibitors and inducers of CYP enzymes and P-glycoprotein. Med Lett Drugs Ther 2017 September 18 (epub). Available at: medicalletter.org/downloads/CYP_PGP_Tables.pdf.

14. BN Wikner et al. Use of benzodiazepines and benzodiazepine receptor agonists during pregnancy: neonatal outcome and congenital malformations. Pharmacoepidemiol Drug Saf 2007; 16:1203.

15. MJ Rapoport et al. Benzodiazepine use and driving: a meta-analysis. J Clin Psychiatry 2009; 70:663.

16. B Albrecht et al. Benzodiazepine use and aggressive behaviour: a systematic review. Aust N Z J Psychiatry 2014; 48:1096.

17. I Hernandez. Exposure-response association between concurrent opioid and benzodiazepine use and risk of opioid-related overdose in Medicare Part D beneficiaries. JAMA Network Open 2018; 1:e180919.

18. ACOG Practice Bulletin: clinical management guidelines for obstetrician-gynecologists number 92, April 2008 (replaces Practice Bulletin number 87, November 2007). Use of psychiatric medications during pregnancy and lactation. Obstet Gynecol 2008; 111:1001.

19. A Kuriyama et al. Ramelteon for the treatment of insomnia in adults: a systematic review and meta-analysis. Sleep Med 2014; 15:385.

20. AD Krystal et al. Efficacy and safety of doxepin 3 and 6 mg in a 35-day sleep laboratory trial in adults with chronic primary insomnia. Sleep 2011; 34:1433.

21. JM Uslaner et al. Orexin receptor antagonists differ from standard sleep drugs by promoting sleep at doses that do not disrupt cognition. Sci Transl Med 2013; 5:179ra44.

22. Suvorexant (Belsomra) for insomnia. Med Lett Drugs Ther 2015; 57:29.

23. A Kuriyama and H Tabata. Suvorexant for the treatment of primary insomnia: a systematic review and meta-analysis. Sleep Med Rev 2017; 35:1.

24. H Sun et al. Effects of suvorexant, an orexin receptor antagonist, on breathing during sleep in patients with chronic obstructive pulmonary disease. Respir Med 2015; 109:416.

25. MH Wiegand. Antidepressants for the treatment of insomnia: a suitable approach? Drugs 2008; 68:2411.

26. WB Mendelson. A review of the evidence for the efficacy and safety of trazodone in insomnia. J Clin Psychiatry 2005; 66:469.

27. ED Hermes et al. Use of second-generation antipsychotic agents for sleep and sedation: a provider survey. Sleep 2013; 36:597.

28. SL Anderson and JP Vande Griend. Quetiapine for insomnia: a review of the literature. Am J Health Syst Pharm 2014; 71:394.

29. T Atkin et al. Drugs for insomnia beyond benzodiazepines: pharmacology, clinical application, and discovery. Pharmacol Rev 2018; 70:197.

30. C Fox et al. Anticholinergic medication use and cognitive impairment in the older population: the medical research council cognitive function and ageing study. J Am Geriatr Soc 2011; 59:1477.

31. AG Wade et al. Nightly treatment of primary insomnia with prolonged release melatonin for 6 months: a randomized placebo controlled trial on age and endogenous melatonin as predictors of efficacy and safety. BMC Med 2010; 8:51.
32. DM Taibi et al. A systematic review of valerian as a sleep aid: safe but not effective. Sleep Med Rev 2007; 11:209.
33. J Sarris and GJ Byrne. A systematic review of insomnia and complementary medicine. Sleep Med Rev 2011; 15:99.

Nonopioid Drugs for Pain

Original publication date – February 2018

Nonopioid drugs can be used in the treatment of many nociceptive and neuropathic pain conditions. Use of opioids for pain will be reviewed in a future issue.

NONOPIOID ANALGESICS

Nonopioid analgesics, unlike full opioid agonists, have a dose ceiling on their analgesic effect.[1]

ACETAMINOPHEN — Acetaminophen has no clinically significant anti-inflammatory activity. It is less effective than full doses of NSAIDs in relieving pain, but has fewer adverse effects. It is available in multiple oral formulations, often in combination with other over-the-counter (OTC) or prescription drugs, and in rectal and intravenous formulations.[2]

Adverse Effects – Most healthy patients can take up to 4 grams of acetaminophen daily with no adverse effects,[3] but repeated use of such doses has been associated with alanine aminotransferase (ALT) elevations.[4] A dosage of 1 gram three times daily for 2 weeks has been shown to increase blood pressure slightly in patients with cardiovascular disease.[5] Acetaminophen overdose can cause serious or fatal hepatotoxicity. In some patients, such as those who are fasting, are heavy alcohol users, or are concurrently taking isoniazid (INH), zidovudine (*Retrovir*, and others),

129

Recommendations for Treatment of Pain

Acute Pain

- For initial treatment of **mild to moderate acute pain**, nonopioid analgesics such as aspirin, acetaminophen, and NSAIDs are preferred.
- For **localized pain**, topical agents, including topical diclofenac, capsaicin, and lidocaine, can be used alone or as adjunctive treatment.
- For **moderate acute pain**, most NSAIDs are more effective than aspirin or acetaminophen and some have equal or greater efficacy compared to oral opioids combined with acetaminophen or even injected opioids.
- For **moderate to severe acute pain**, a combination of an NSAID and acetaminophen may be as effective as an opioid/acetaminophen combination.
- For **severe acute pain,** immediate-release formulations of full opioid agonists are the drugs of choice.

Chronic Noncancer Pain

- Nonpharmacologic therapy and nonopioid pharmacologic therapy are recommended for treatment of chronic noncancer pain.
- Nonpharmacologic therapies that have shown efficacy for treatment of chronic pain include structured education and exercise programs, cognitive behavioral therapy, acupuncture, meditation, and massage.
- NSAIDs are more effective than acetaminophen, but long-term use can result in serious adverse effects including gastrointestinal, renal, and cardiovascular toxicity.
- For severe chronic pain that has not responded to other agents, use of opioids may be necessary.

Chronic Cancer Pain

- Full opioid agonists are generally the drugs of choice for severe chronic cancer pain.

Neuropathic Pain

- For initial treatment of neuropathic pain, an antidepressant or an antiepileptic can be used.
- Topical agents such as lidocaine and capsaicin can be used for localized neuropathic pain.
- Combining an antidepressant and an antiepileptic may produce a synergistic analgesic effect in neuropathic pain syndromes.
- For severe pain that has not responded to other agents, use of opioids may be necessary.

or a barbiturate, hepatotoxicity can develop after moderate overdosage or even with high therapeutic doses. Continued use of acetaminophen may increase the anticoagulant effect of warfarin (*Coumadin*, and others) in some patients.[6] Some meta-analyses of cohort and case-control studies have suggested that long-term use of acetaminophen may increase the risk of developing renal cell cancer.[7]

Pregnancy – Occasional use of oral acetaminophen during pregnancy is generally considered safe.

SALICYLATES — **Aspirin** is effective for most types of mild to moderate pain, but it is now used mainly in low doses as a platelet inhibitor. Unlike other NSAIDs, a single dose of aspirin irreversibly inhibits platelet function for the 8- to 10-day life of the platelet, interfering with hemostasis and prolonging bleeding time.

Adverse Effects – A single dose of aspirin can precipitate asthma symptoms in aspirin-sensitive patients. High doses or chronic use of aspirin can cause gastrointestinal (GI) ulceration and salicylate intoxication. Taking buffered or enteric-coated formulations can reduce GI upset but not the risk of GI ulceration, and could delay pain relief. Aspirin should not be used during viral syndromes in children and teenagers because of the risk of Reye's syndrome.

Salsalate and diflunisal are nonacetylated salicylates. Salsalate does not interfere with platelet aggregation. Although low doses (250 mg twice daily) of diflunisal have no effect on platelets and the usual dosage of 500 mg twice daily has a minimal effect that is not likely to have clinical significance, a dosage of 1000 mg twice daily, which is larger than the recommended maximum dosage, may transiently inhibit platelet function.[62] These drugs are rarely associated with GI bleeding, and are well tolerated by asthmatic patients, but there are no controlled trials demonstrating their comparative efficacy for treatment of chronic pain.

Table 1. Some Nonopioid Analgesics for Pain

Drug	Some Available Formulations
Acetaminophen[3] – generic *Tylenol* (McNeil Consumer)	325, 500 mg tabs[4]
Ofirmev (Mallinckrodt)	10 mg/mL IV soln
Salicylates	
Aspirin – generic *Bayer* (Bayer)	325 mg tabs, 500 mg caplets[4,8]
Diflunisal – generic	500 mg tabs
Salsalate – generic	500, 750 mg tabs
Some Nonselective NSAIDs	
Diclofenac[9] – generic	50 mg tabs
Dyloject (Hospira) *Zipsor* (Depomed) *Zorvolex* (Iroko)	37.5 mg/mL single-dose vials 25 mg caps 18, 35 mg caps

1. Dosage adjustment may be needed for renal or hepatic impairment.
2. Approximate WAC for one week of treatment with the lowest dose and/or longest dosing interval. WAC = wholesaler acquisition cost or manufacturer's published price to wholesalers; WAC represents a published catalogue or list price and may not represent an actual transactional price. Source: AnalySource® Monthly. January 5, 2018. Reprinted with permission by First Databank, Inc. All rights reserved. ©2018. www.fdbhealth.com/policies/drug-pricing-policy.
3. Acetaminophen is included in multiple prescription and OTC products for treatment of pain, cough, cold, flu, migraine, insomnia, etc., increasing the risk for accidental overdosage.
4. Also available in other strengths and dosage forms, alone and in combination with other drugs, both OTC and by prescription.

Usual Adult Analgesic Dosage[1]	Comments	Cost[2]
650 mg q4-6h or 1000 mg q6-8h (max 4000 mg/d)	Less effective than full doses of NSAIDs Amount in prescription combination products limited to 325 mg/dosage unit	$1.30[5] 4.20[5]
<50 kg: 15 mg/kg q6h or 12.5 mg/kg q4h (max 75 mg/kg/d) ≥50 kg: 1000 mg q6h or 650 mg q4h (max 4000 mg/d)		112.60[6,7]
325-650 mg q4-6h (max 4000 mg/d)		0.30[5] 1.70[5]
500 mg q8-12h (max 1500 mg/d)	500 mg comparable to 650 mg of acetaminophen or aspirin with slower onset and longer duration	79.00
500 mg q6h or 1000 mg q12h (max 3000 mg/d)		33.30
50 mg q8-12h (max 200 mg/d)	Comparable to aspirin with longer duration	14.60
37.5 mg IV q6h (max 150 mg/d)	Also available in a fixed-dose combination with misoprostol (Arthrotec) to decrease GI toxicity	63.00[7]
25 mg qid (max 200 mg/d)		303.40
18 or 35 mg tid		81.70

5. Cost at www.walgreens.com. Accessed February 1, 2018.
6. Cost based on treatment of a 70-kg patient.
7. Cost for one day of treatment at the lowest dosage.
8. Also available in chewable, buffered, enteric-coated, and extended-release formulations.
9. Also available in enteric-coated and extended-release tabs for use in osteoarthritis, rheumatoid arthritis, and ankylosing spondylitis, as a topical patch (Flector) for treatment of pain due to minor strains, sprains, and contusions, as a topical gel (Voltaren 1% Gel) for use in osteoarthritis, and as a topical solution (Pennsaid 2%) for use in osteoarthritis of the knee.

Continued on next page

Table 1. Some Nonopioid Analgesics for Pain (continued)

Drug	Some Available Formulations
Some Nonselective NSAIDs (continued)	
Etodolac – generic	200, 300 mg caps; 400, 500 mg tabs
extended-release – generic[11]	400, 500, 600 mg ER tabs
Fenoprofen – generic	200, 400 mg caps; 600 mg tabs
Nalfon (Xspire)	400 mg caps
Flurbiprofen[11] – generic	50, 100 mg tabs
Ibuprofen – generic	400, 600, 800 mg tabs
Caldolor (Cumberland)	100 mg/mL IV soln
Ibuprofen OTC – generic *Advil* (Pfizer Consumer)	100, 200 mg tabs; 200 mg caps
Ketoprofen – generic	50, 75 mg caps
extended-release – generic	200 mg ER caps

ER = extended-release
10. For use in osteoarthritis or rheumatoid arthritis the dosage is 300 mg bid or tid, 400 mg bid, or 500 mg bid.

Usual Adult Analgesic Dosage[1]	Comments	Cost[2]
200-400 mg q6-8h (max 1000 mg/d)[10]	200 mg comparable to ibuprofen 400 mg; possibly	$4.90
400-1000 mg once/d	superior to aspirin 650 mg	16.20
200 mg q4-6h (max 3200 mg/d)[12]		333.50
		96.20[13]
100 mg q12h (max 300 mg/d)		5.90
400 mg q4-6h (max 2400 mg/d)	200 mg equal to 650 mg of aspirin or acetaminophen; 400 mg comparable to acetaminophen/codeine Also available in a fixed-dose combination with famotidine (Duexis) to decrease GI toxicity	3.80
400-800 mg IV q6h (max 3200 mg/d)	Modest opioid-sparing effect Effectiveness compared to IV ketorolac unclear	29.40[7]
200-400 mg q4-6h (max 1200 mg/d)	200 mg equal to 650 mg of aspirin or acetaminophen	1.10[5] 2.20[5]
50 mg q6h or 75 mg q8h (max 300 mg/d)	25 mg comparable to ibuprofen 400 mg and superior to aspirin 650 mg; 50 mg superior to acetaminophen/codeine combination	14.10
200 mg once/d		60.60

11. FDA-approved only for use in osteoarthritis and rheumatoid arthritis.
12. For use in osteoarthritis or rheumatoid arthritis, the dosage is 400-600 mg tid or qid.
13. Cost for one week of treatment with 400 mg tid.

Continued on next page

Table 1. Some Nonopioid Analgesics for Pain (continued)

Drug	Some Available Formulations
Some Nonselective NSAIDs (continued)	
Ketorolac – generic	10 mg tabs
	15 mg/mL, 30 mg/mL, 60 mg/2 mL injection
Sprix (Egalet)	15.75 mg/intranasal spray
Meclofenamate – generic	50, 100 mg caps
Mefenamic acid – generic	250 mg caps
Meloxicam – generic[11]	7.5, 15 mg tabs; 7.5 mg/5 mL PO susp
Mobic (Boehringer Ingelheim)[11]	7.5, 15 mg tabs
Vivlodex (Iroko)[21]	5, 10 mg caps
Nabumetone[11] – generic	500, 750 mg tabs
Naproxen – generic	250, 375, 500 mg tabs; 375, 500 mg enteric-coated tabs; 25 mg/mL PO susp
Naprosyn, EC-Naprosyn (Canton, Key)	500 mg tabs; 375, 500 mg enteric-coated tabs; 25 mg/mL PO susp

14. Recommended only for continuation therapy after IM or IV ketorolac; total use of ketorolac not to exceed 5 days.
15. Cost of 5 days' treatment.
16. Use should be limited to 5 days because of GI toxicity; can also be given IM as a single 60 mg (<65 yrs) or 30 mg (≥65 years) dose.
17. Cost of 5 days' treatment for a <65-year-old patient.

Usual Adult Analgesic Dosage[1]	Comments	Cost[2]
10 mg q4-6h (max 40 mg/d)[14]	10 mg comparable to ibuprofen 400 or 800 mg or naproxen 500-550 mg	$28.50[15]
<65 yrs: 30 mg IM or IV q6h (max 120 mg/d)[16] >65 yrs: 15 mg IM or IV q6h (max 60 mg/d)[16]	Comparable to 12 mg IM morphine with longer duration	30.20[17]
<65 yrs: 1 spray q6-8h in each nostril (max 126 mg/d)[18] >65 yrs: 1 spray q6-8h in one nostril (max 63 mg/d)[18]		1625.70[19]
50-100 mg q4h (max 400 mg/d)		140.10
500 mg once, then 250 mg q6h[20] (max 1250 mg d 1, then 1000 mg/d)	Comparable to aspirin but more effective in dysmenorrhea	93.20
7.5-15 mg once/d	Appears to be more selective for COX-2 than COX-1 at low doses (7.5 mg)	0.70 54.70
5 or 10 mg once/d		167.40
500 or 750 mg q8-12h (max 2000 mg/d)		16.10
250 mg q6-8h or 500 mg q12h (max 1250 mg d 1, then 1000 mg/d)	250 mg probably comparable to aspirin 650 mg with longer duration; 500 mg superior to aspirin 650 mg	2.30 83.00

18. Dose in patients weighing <50 kg or with renal impairment (GFR 30-90 mL/min) is one spray in one nostril; maximum 4 doses/day for up to 5 days.
19. Cost of one carton containing 5 single-day nasal spray bottles.
20. Duration of use usually not to exceed 1 week for acute pain or 2-3 days for dysmenorrhea.
21. FDA-approved only for use in osteoarthritis.

Continued on next page

Table 1. Some Nonopioid Analgesics for Pain (continued)	
Drug	**Some Available Formulations**
Some Nonselective NSAIDs (continued)	
Naproxen sodium –	
generic	275, 550 mg tabs
Anaprox DS (Canton)	550 mg tabs
Naproxen sodium OTC –	
generic	220 mg tabs
Aleve (Bayer)	
Selective COX-2 Inhibitor	
Celecoxib – generic	50, 100, 200, 400 mg caps
Celebrex (Pfizer)	

22. The dosage is 200 mg/d for use in osteoarthritis and 200-400 mg/d for use in rheumatoid arthritis.

NSAIDS — Single full doses of nonselective NSAIDs such as ibuprofen or naproxen are more effective than full doses of acetaminophen or aspirin for treatment of acute pain.[8] Some NSAIDs have an analgesic effect that is equal to or greater than that of usual doses of an oral opioid combined with acetaminophen.[9] Intramuscular or intravenous ketorolac is comparable in analgesic efficacy to moderate doses of morphine in patients with acute pain. An IV formulation of diclofenac *(Dyloject)* may act more rapidly than IV ketorolac, but is otherwise similar in efficacy.[10]

How NSAIDs compare to other analgesics for treatment of chronic pain is less well established. Some patients may respond better to one NSAID than another. The COX-2-selective NSAID celecoxib is about

Usual Adult Analgesic Dosage[1]	Comments	Cost[2]
275 mg q6-8h or 550 mg q12h (max 1375 mg d 1, then 1100 mg/d)	275 mg comparable to aspirin 650 mg with longer duration; 550 mg superior to aspirin 650 mg with longer duration Also available in a fixed-dose combination with esomeprazole (Vimovo) to decrease GI toxicity	$10.50 130.30
220 mg q8-12h (max 660 mg/d)	440 mg comparable to 400 mg ibuprofen with longer duration	1.30[5] 1.70[5]
400 mg once, then 200 mg q12h (max 600 mg d 1, then 400 mg/d)[22]	Less effective than full doses of naproxen or ibuprofen	16.10 168.80

as effective as a nonselective NSAID for treatment of osteoarthritis and rheumatoid arthritis,[11] but it is less effective for treatment of acute pain, such as that following surgical or dental procedures.

Low-dose oral formulations of three NSAIDs, diclofenac (Zorvolex), indomethacin (Tivorbex), and meloxicam (Vivlodex), have been approved by the FDA for treatment of mild to moderate acute pain and/or osteoarthritis pain. They are formulated as submicron particles that increase surface area, leading to faster dissolution and absorption. How they compare in efficacy and safety to standard doses of the same drugs, which cost much less, is unknown.[12-14] The potent NSAID indomethacin is associated with a high risk of adverse effects; it should not be used in any dosage for treatment of mild to moderate pain.

Guidelines from the American College of Physicians recommend NSAIDs as first-line options for patients with chronic low back pain who have an inadequate response to nonpharmacologic treatment.[15] Meta-analyses of randomized trials in patients with chronic low back pain or spinal pain have found that NSAIDs reduce pain intensity and improve disability compared to placebo; the efficacy of different NSAIDs appeared to be similar in these patients.[16,17]

Bleeding – All NSAIDs, except celecoxib and, to a lesser extent, meloxicam and nabumetone, can interfere with platelet function and prolong bleeding time. The NSAID-induced antiplatelet effect, unlike that of aspirin, is reversible when the NSAID is cleared.

GI Adverse Effects – Dyspepsia and GI ulceration, perforation, and bleeding can occur with all NSAIDs, including parenteral formulations, often without warning. High doses, prolonged use, previous peptic ulcer disease, concomitant systemic corticosteroids or aspirin (even 81 mg/day), excessive alcohol intake, and advanced age increase the risk of these complications. Use of ketorolac is limited to 5 days because of its high risk of GI toxicity. Celecoxib appears to cause less GI toxicity than nonselective NSAIDs.[18]

Taking an NSAID with a proton pump inhibitor such as omeprazole (*Prilosec OTC*, and generics), an H2-receptor antagonist such as ranitidine (*Zantac*, and generics), or the prostaglandin analog misoprostol (*Cytotec*, and generics) may decrease the incidence of GI toxicity.[19] *Arthrotec* (diclofenac/misoprostol), *Vimovo* (naproxen/esomeprazole), and *Duexis* (ibuprofen/famotidine) are three commercially-available combinations of an NSAID and a gastroprotective agent.[20,21]

Renal Toxicity – All NSAIDs, including celecoxib, inhibit renal prostaglandins, decrease renal blood flow, cause fluid retention, and may cause hypertension and renal failure, particularly in elderly patients. Diminished renal function or decreased effective intravascular volume due to diuretic therapy, cirrhosis, or heart failure can increase the risk of NSAID-induced renal toxicity.

Cardiovascular Effects – An increased risk of serious cardiovascular events, including myocardial infarction, stroke, and out-of-hospital cardiac arrest has been reported with some NSAIDs; the risk appears to be highest with diclofenac and lowest with naproxen.[22-24]

In one randomized trial in patients with osteoarthritis or rheumatoid arthritis and cardiovascular risk factors, celecoxib was found to be noninferior to the nonselective NSAIDs ibuprofen and naproxen with regard to cardiovascular safety.[25] However, the average dose of celecoxib (about 200 mg/day) was lower than the doses previously associated with cardiotoxicity. In addition, about 50% of the patients were taking low-dose aspirin at baseline; since ibuprofen and naproxen, but not celecoxib, inhibit aspirin binding to platelet COX-1, the cardioprotective effects of aspirin may have been blunted in patients who took ibuprofen or naproxen.[26]

Other Effects – Like aspirin, nonaspirin NSAIDs can precipitate asthma symptoms and anaphylactoid reactions in aspirin-sensitive patients. They frequently cause small increases in aminotransferase levels; serious hepatotoxicity is rare, but may occur more frequently with diclofenac. Pancreatitis has been reported. Cholestatic hepatitis has occurred with celecoxib.

NSAIDs can cause CNS adverse effects such as dizziness, anxiety, drowsiness, confusion, depression, disorientation, severe headache, and aseptic meningitis. They have been associated with both mild and severe skin reactions, including exfoliative dermatitis, Stevens-Johnson syndrome, and toxic epidermal necrolysis. NSAIDs rarely cause blood dyscrasias; aplastic anemia has been reported with ibuprofen, fenoprofen, naproxen, indomethacin, tolmetin, and piroxicam. Long-term use of nonaspirin NSAIDs has been associated with an increased risk of renal cell cancer.[27]

Pregnancy – Exposure to NSAIDs during pregnancy or around the time of conception has been associated with an increased risk of miscarriage, but the data are weak. Use of NSAIDs during the third trimester of pregnancy may cause premature closure of the ductus arteriosus and persistent pulmonary hypertension in the neonate, but these effects appear to be uncommon if the drug is discontinued 6-8 weeks before delivery.

Drug Interactions – NSAIDs can decrease the effectiveness of diuretics, beta blockers, ACE inhibitors, and some other antihypertensive drugs, and can increase serum concentrations of lithium and methotrexate, possibly resulting in toxicity. They may increase the INR in patients taking warfarin. Patients taking aspirin for cardiovascular protection should not take ibuprofen or naproxen regularly because they can interfere with aspirin's antiplatelet effect.

COMBINATION TREATMENT FOR ACUTE PAIN — A combination of an NSAID and acetaminophen is more effective than either drug alone and may be an alternative to opioid analgesics for treatment of moderate to severe acute pain. In a double-blind trial, 411 patients with moderate to severe acute extremity pain were randomized to treatment with single doses of one of four combination analgesic regimens (ibuprofen 400 mg plus acetaminophen 1000 mg or either oxycodone 5 mg, hydrocodone 5 mg, or codeine 30 mg plus acetaminophen 300-325 mg). There were no statistically significant differences in pain reduction between the nonopioid regimen and the opioid-containing regimens at two hours after administration of the drugs.[28]

ADJUVANT PAIN MEDICATIONS

Antidepressants and antiepileptics are the mainstay of treatment for a variety of **neuropathic pain** syndromes, including postherpetic neuralgia, diabetic neuropathy, fibromyalgia, complex regional pain syndrome, and phantom limb pain, even though most of them are not FDA-approved for these indications.

ANTIDEPRESSANTS — Tricyclic antidepressants such as **amitriptyline**, **nortriptyline**, and **imipramine** can relieve many types of neuropathic pain, including diabetic neuropathy, postherpetic neuralgia, polyneuropathy, and nerve injury or infiltration with cancer. They are also effective for treatment of fibromyalgia pain.[29] The analgesic effects of these drugs are likely due to their inhibition of norepinephrine and serotonin reuptake. They commonly cause orthostatic hypotension, weight gain, sedation, sexual dysfunction, and anticholinergic effects (urinary retention, constipation, dry mouth, blurred vision, memory impairment, and confusion).

Venlafaxine, a serotonin and norepinephrine reuptake inhibitor (SNRI), has been reported to be effective in various types of neuropathic pain, including diabetic neuropathy, post-mastectomy pain syndrome, and chemotherapy-induced neurotoxicity, and has also been used to treat fibromyalgia,[30,31] but it is not FDA-approved for any of these indications. **Duloxetine**, another SNRI, is FDA-approved for treatment of pain associated with diabetic peripheral neuropathy and fibromyalgia, and for chronic musculoskeletal pain.[32-34] In patients with chronic low back pain or osteoarthritis, it is only modestly more effective than placebo. **Milnacipran**, an SNRI approved by the FDA only for use in fibromyalgia,[35] is moderately effective in decreasing pain and improving function. It inhibits norepinephrine reuptake to a greater extent than it does serotonin reuptake. How it compares to venlafaxine or duloxetine is unclear. SNRIs can cause nausea, dizziness, increased sweating, tachycardia, constipation, urinary retention, and a dose-dependent increase in blood pressure. Severe discontinuation symptoms and sustained hypertension can occur with venlafaxine. Severe liver injury has been reported with duloxetine and milnacipran.

There is no good evidence that selective serotonin reuptake inhibitors (SSRIs) are effective for treatment of neuropathic pain.[36]

ANTIEPILEPTICS — In controlled trials, **gabapentin** has been effective in reducing pain in postherpetic neuralgia (an FDA-approved use) and diabetic neuropathy.[37] Gabapentin can cause dizziness, somnolence, peripheral edema, and weight gain. **Pregabalin**, which is similar in structure to gabapentin, is now available in a once-daily, extended-release

Table 2. Some Adjuvant Pain Medications[1]

Drug	Some Available Formulations
Tricyclic Antidepressants	
Amitriptyline – generic	10, 25, 50, 75, 100, 150 mg tabs
Imipramine HCl – generic *Tofranil* (Mallinckrodt)	10, 25, 50 mg tabs
Imipramine pamoate – generic	75, 100, 125, 150 mg caps
Nortriptyline – generic *Pamelor* (Mallinckrodt)	10, 25, 50, 75 mg caps; 10 mg/5 mL PO soln 10, 25, 50, 75 mg caps
Serotonin and Norepinephrine Reuptake Inhibitors (SNRIs)	

Venlafaxine – generic
  extended-release – generic
  Effexor XR (Pfizer)
	25, 37.5, 50, 75, 100 mg tabs
	37.5, 75, 150 tabs and caps; 225 mg tabs
	37.5, 75, 150 mg caps

Duloxetine – generic *Cymbalta* (Lilly)	20, 30, 60 mg delayed-release caps
Milnacipran – *Savella* (Allergan)	12.5, 25, 50, 100 mg tabs
Antiepileptics	

Gabapentin – generic
  Neurontin (Pfizer)
  extended-release
  Gralise (Depomed)
  Horizant (GlaxoSmithKline)
	100, 300, 400 mg caps; 600, 800 mg tabs;
	  250 mg/5 mL PO soln
	
	300, 600 mg ER tabs
	600 mg ER tabs

Pregabalin – *Lyrica* (Pfizer)
 	
  extended-release – *Lyrica CR*
	25, 50, 75, 100, 150, 200, 225, 300 mg caps;
	  20 mg/mL PO soln
	82.5, 165, 330 mg ER tabs

Carbamazepine – generic
  Tegretol (Novartis)
  extended-release – generic
 	
  Tegretol XR
  Carbatrol (Shire)
  Equetro (Validus)
	200 mg tabs; 100 mg chewable tabs;
	  100 mg/5 mL PO susp
	100, 200 mg ER caps and tabs; 300 mg ER
	  caps; 400 mg ER tabs
	100, 200, 400 mg ER tabs
	100, 200, 300 mg ER caps
	100, 200, 300 mg ER caps

ER = extended-release
1. Some of the drugs listed here are not FDA-approved for treatment of pain.
2. Dosage may need to be adjusted for renal or hepatic impairment.
3. Approximate WAC for 30 days' treatment at the lowest usual dosage and/or longest dosing interval.
   WAC = wholesaler acquisition cost or manufacturer's published price to wholesalers; WAC represents
   a published catalogue or list price and may not represent an actual transactional price. Source:
   AnalySource® Monthly. January 5, 2018. Reprinted with permission by First Databank, Inc. All rights
   reserved. ©2018. www.fdbhealth.com/policies/drug-pricing-policy.

Usual Dosage for Pain[2]	Cost[3]
25-100 mg once/d	$8.50
50-100 mg once/d or divided	15.40
	613.20
75-100 mg once/d	354.00
75 mg once/d or divided	13.50
	1249.60
75 mg once/d-tid	10.70
75-150 mg once/d	15.70
	422.20
60 mg once/d	19.30
	239.70
50 mg bid	348.80
600-1200 mg tid	14.30
	908.60
1800 mg once/d	695.00
600 mg bid	777.00
75-300 mg bid or 50-200 mg tid	445.00
330-660 mg once/d	383.10
200-400 mg bid	53.70
	143.40
200-400 mg bid	201.80
	153.20
	106.40
	217.90

Continued on next page

Table 2. Some Adjuvant Pain Medications[1] (continued)	
Drug	**Some Available Formulations**
Antiepileptics (continued)	
Oxcarbazepine – generic *Trileptal* (Novartis) extended-release	150, 300, 600 mg tabs; 300 mg/5 mL PO susp
Oxtellar XR (Supernus)	150, 300, 600 mg ER tabs
ER = extended-release	

formulation. Immediate-release and extended-release pregabalin are FDA-approved for treatment of postherpetic neuralgia and diabetic peripheral neuropathy. The immediate-release formulation is also approved for fibromyalgia (the extended-release formulation failed to show efficacy in these patients).[38,39] In a randomized, double-blind, 8-week trial in 209 patients with acute or chronic sciatica, pregabalin 150-600 mg daily did not significantly reduce the intensity of leg pain compared to placebo.[40] The dose of pregabalin can be titrated more rapidly than that of gabapentin. Like gabapentin, it can cause dizziness, somnolence, and peripheral edema; significant weight gain has been reported in some patients.

Use of higher-than-recommended doses of gabapentin and pregabalin to achieve euphoric highs is increasingly being reported; risk factors include a history of substance abuse, particularly of opioids, and the presence of psychiatric comorbidities.[41,42] Pregabalin is a schedule V controlled substance.

Carbamazepine is FDA-approved for treatment of pain due to trigeminal neuralgia. **Oxcarbazepine**, which is structurally related to carbamazepine, is not FDA-approved for treatment of pain. It has been shown to be modestly effective in relieving peripheral neuropathic pain, and may be better tolerated than carbamazepine.[43]

COMBINATION TREATMENT FOR NEUROPATHIC PAIN — Combining an antidepressant and an antiepileptic may produce a synergistic

Usual Dosage for Pain[2]	Cost[3]
300-600 mg bid	$33.00
	494.00
600-2400 mg once/d	470.90

analgesic effect in neuropathic pain syndromes, but clinical trials have produced conflicting results. In one study in patients with diabetic polyneuropathy or postherpetic neuralgia, a combination of gabapentin and nortriptyline was more effective than monotherapy with either drug alone.[44] However, in another study in patients with diabetic peripheral neuropathy, a combination of standard doses of pregabalin and duloxetine was not significantly different from high-dose monotherapy with either drug alone.[45]

In a study in patients with neuropathic pain, taking lower doses of gabapentin and morphine together provided better analgesia than taking either drug alone.[46] However, a population-based, case-control study found that opioid users taking moderate or high doses of gabapentin concomitantly had a significantly increased risk of opioid-related death.[47]

OTHER DRUGS — Ziconotide *(Prialt)*, a synthetic neuronal N-type calcium channel blocker, is administered intrathecally via a programmable microinfusion device for treatment of severe chronic pain. The drug has been effective, both as monotherapy and when added to standard therapy, for treatment of refractory severe chronic pain, including neuropathic pain. Severe psychiatric effects (paranoid reactions, psychosis) and CNS toxicity (confusion, somnolence, unresponsiveness) can occur. Use of a low starting dose followed by titration in small increments once weekly is recommended to increase tolerability.[48,49] Unlike opioids, ziconotide does not cause tolerance, dependence, or respiratory depression, and is not a controlled substance.[50]

Caffeine in doses of 65-200 mg may enhance the analgesic effect of acetaminophen, aspirin, or ibuprofen in patients with acute pain.[51] **Hydroxyzine** given parenterally in doses of 25-50 mg may add to the analgesic effect of opioids in postoperative and cancer pain while reducing the incidence of nausea and vomiting. **Corticosteroids** can produce analgesia in some patients with inflammatory diseases or tumor infiltration of nerves. The oral and transdermal patch formulations of the alpha$_2$-adrenergic agonist **clonidine** may improve pain and hyperalgesia in sympathetically maintained pain, but can cause hypotension. Injections of **botulinum toxin type A** have been shown to be effective for treatment of postherpetic neuralgia, diabetic neuropathy, trigeminal neuralgia, and intractable neuropathic pain such as poststroke pain and spinal cord injury.[52]

Cannabis and Cannabinoids – Two oral prescription cannabinoids are available in the US. **Dronabinol** (*Marinol*, and generics), a synthetic form of delta-9 tetrahydrocannabinol (THC), and **nabilone** *(Cesamet)*, a synthetic analog of THC, are both FDA-approved for treatment of nausea and vomiting associated with cancer chemotherapy; dronabinol is also approved for anorexia in patients with AIDS. Use of cannabis and cannabinoids for treatment of pain remains controversial. Randomized trials of cannabinoids have found some evidence of efficacy for second-line treatment of cancer pain, neuropathic pain, and the spasticity of multiple sclerosis, but none are currently approved by the FDA for these indications.[53] Results of randomized controlled trials of cannabis products, including nabiximols, a standardized cannabis extract available outside the US, suggest that cannabis may alleviate neuropathic pain over the short term in some patients; the efficacy of cannabis for other types of chronic pain remains to be established.[54,55]

Topical Analgesics – A 5% **lidocaine** patch *(Lidoderm)* is FDA-approved for treatment of postherpetic neuralgia.[56] It is widely used off-label for other types of pain despite a lack of clinical trials supporting its efficacy. Skin irritation can occur at the site of application. An 8% **capsaicin** patch *(Qutenza)* is FDA-approved for treatment of postherpetic neuralgia.[57] Application of the patch for one hour is modestly effective in reducing pain associated with postherpetic neuralgia for up to 3 months. The patch is applied during an office visit; an increase in pain is common during and for a few days after application. Topical **diclofenac** is available as a patch *(Flector)*, a gel *(Voltaren 1%)* and a solution *(Pennsaid 2%)* for treatment of osteoarthritis or musculoskeletal pain.

Topical analgesics containing menthol, methylsalicylate, or capsaicin are available OTC for treatment of mild muscle and joint pain; while generally well-tolerated, there have been rare reports of severe skin burns requiring treatment or hospitalization.[58] A 4% lidocaine patch is also available OTC.

NONPHARMACOLOGIC THERAPIES — Some nonpharmacologic therapies that have shown efficacy for treatment of chronic pain include structured education and exercise programs, cognitive behavioral therapy, acupuncture, meditation, and massage.[59] Movement therapies such as yoga, pilates, and tai chi may also be effective.[60] A large review of clinical studies examining exercise programs for various types of chronic pain found that these interventions are unlikely to cause harm and may be associated with improvements in pain severity and physical function.[61] Guidelines from the American College of Physicians recommend nonpharmacologic therapies as a first-line option for treatment of low back pain.[17]

1. DE Becker et al. Pain management: Part 1: Managing acute and postoperative dental pain. Anesth Prog 2010; 57:67.
2. Intravenous acetaminophen (Ofirmev). Med Lett Drugs Ther 2011; 53:26.
3. Acetaminophen safety - Deja vu. Med Lett Drugs Ther 2009; 51:53.
4. PB Watkins et al. Aminotransferase elevations in healthy adults receiving 4 grams of acetaminophen daily: a randomized controlled trial. JAMA 2006; 296:87.
5. In brief: Does acetaminophen increase blood pressure? Med Lett Drugs Ther 2011; 53:29.
6. Addendum: Warfarin-acetaminophen interaction. Med Lett Drugs Ther 2008; 50:45.
7. S Karami et al. Analgesic use and risk of renal cell carcinoma: a case-control, cohort and meta-analytic assessment. Int J Cancer 2016; 139:584.
8. JA Forbes et al. Evaluation of bromfenac, aspirin, and ibuprofen in postoperative oral surgery pain. Pharmacotherapy 1991; 11:64.
9. M Nauta et al. Codeine-acetaminophen versus nonsteroidal anti-inflammatory drugs in the treatment of post-abdominal surgery pain: a systematic review of randomized trials. Am J Surg 2009; 198:256.

10. Intravenous diclofenac (Dyloject). Med Lett Drugs Ther 2015; 57:171.
11. PL McCormack. Celecoxib: a review of its use for symptomatic relief in the treatment of osteoarthritis, rheumatoid arthritis and ankylosing spondylitis. Drugs 2011; 71:2457.
12. Low-dose diclofenac (Zorvolex) for pain. Med Lett Drugs Ther 2014; 56:19.
13. In brief: Low-dose indomethacin (Tivorbex) for pain. Med Lett Drugs Ther 2014; 56:64.
14. Low-dose meloxicam (Vivlodex) for osteoarthritis pain. Med Lett Drugs Ther 2016; 58:35.
15. WT Enthoven et al. Non-steroidal anti-inflammatory drugs for chronic low back pain. Cochrane Database Syst Rev 2016; 2:CD012087.
16. GC Machado et al. Non-steroidal anti-inflammatory drugs for spinal pain: a systematic review and meta-analysis. Ann Rheum Dis 2017; 76:1269.
17. A Qaseem et al. Noninvasive treatments for acute, subacute, and chronic low back pain: a clinical practice guideline from the American College of Physicians. Ann Intern Med 2017; 166:514.
18. FKL Chan et al. Gastrointestinal safety of celecoxib versus naproxen in patients with cardiothrombotic diseases and arthritis after upper gastrointestinal bleeding (CONCERN): an industry-independent, double-blind, double-dummy, randomised trial. Lancet 2017; 389:2375.
19. Primary prevention of ulcers in patients taking aspirin or NSAIDs. Med Lett Drugs Ther 2010; 52:17.
20. Naproxen/esomeprazole (Vimovo). Med Lett Drugs Ther 2010; 52:74.
21. A fixed-dose combination of ibuprofen and famotidine (Duexis). Med Lett Drugs Ther 2011; 53:85.
22. S Trelle et al. Cardiovascular safety of non-steroidal anti-inflammatory drugs: network meta-analysis. BMJ 2011; 342:c7086.
23. P McGettigan and D Henry. Cardiovascular risk with non-steroidal anti-inflammatory drugs: systematic review of population-based controlled observational studies. PLoS Med 2011; 8:e1001098.
24. KB Sondergaard et al. Non-steroidal anti-inflammatory drug use is associated with increased risk of out-of-hospital cardiac arrest: a nationwide case-time-control study. Eur Heart J Cardiovasc Pharmacother 2017; 3:100.
25. SE Nissen et al. Cardiovascular safety of celecoxib, naproxen, or ibuprofen for arthritis. N Engl J Med 2016; 375:2519.
26. Celecoxib safety revisited. Med Lett Drugs Ther 2016; 58:159.
27. TK Choueiri et al. Analgesic use and the risk of kidney cancer: a meta-analysis of epidemiologic studies. Int J Cancer 2014; 134:384.
28. AK Chang et al. Effect of a single dose of oral opioid and nonopioid analgesics on acute extremity pain in the emergency department: a randomized clinical trial. JAMA 2017; 318:1661.
29. W Häuser et al. The role of antidepressants in the management of fibromyalgia syndrome: a systematic review and meta-analysis. CNS Drugs 2012; 26:297.
30. R Aiyer et al. Treatment of neuropathic pain with venlafaxine: a systematic review. Pain Med 2017; 18:1999.
31. LA VanderWeide et al. A systematic review of the efficacy of venlafaxine for the treatment of fibromyalgia. J Clin Pharm Ther 2015; 40:1.

32. Duloxetine (Cymbalta) for diabetic neuropathic pain. Med Lett Drugs Ther 2005; 47:67.
33. Duloxetine (Cymbalta) for fibromyalgia. Med Lett Drugs Ther 2008; 50:57.
34. Duloxetine (Cymbalta) for chronic musculoskeletal pain. Med Lett Drugs Ther 2011; 53:33.
35. Milnacipran (Savella) for fibromyalgia. Med Lett Drugs Ther 2009; 51:45.
36. NB Finnerup et al. Pharmacotherapy for neuropathic pain in adults: a systematic review and meta-analysis. Lancet Neurol 2015; 14:162.
37. Gabapentin (Neurontin) for chronic pain. Med Lett Drugs Ther 2004; 46:29.
38. Pregabalin (Lyrica) for neuropathic pain and epilepsy. Med Lett Drugs Ther 2005; 47:75.
39. W Häuser et al. Treatment of fibromyalgia syndrome with gabapentin and pregabalin—a meta-analysis of randomized controlled trials. Pain 2009; 145:69.
40. S Mathieson et al. Trial of pregabalin for acute and chronic sciatica. N Engl J Med 2017; 376:1111.
41. KE Evoy et al. Abuse and misuse of pregabalin and gabapentin. Drugs 2017; 77:403.
42. GC Quintero. Review about gabapentin misuse, interactions, contraindications and side effects. J Exp Pharmacol 2017; 9:13.
43. M Zhou et al. Oxcarbazepine for neuropathic pain. Cochrane Database Syst Rev 2017; 12:CD007963.
44. I Gilron et al. Nortriptyline and gabapentin, alone and in combination for neuropathic pain: a double-blind, randomised controlled crossover trial. Lancet 2009; 374:1252.
45. S Tesfaye et al. Duloxetine and pregabalin: high-dose monotherapy or their combination? The "COMBO-DN study"—a multinational, randomized, double-blind, parallel-group study in patients with diabetic peripheral neuropathic pain. Pain 2013; 154:2616.
46. I Gilron et al. Morphine, gabapentin, or their combination for neuropathic pain. N Engl J Med 2005; 352:1324.
47. T Gomes et al. Gabapentin, opioids, and the risk of opioid-related death: a population-based nested case-control study. PLoS Med 2017; 14:e1002396.
48. M Sanford. Intrathecal ziconotide: a review of its use in patients with chronic pain refractory to other systemic or intrathecal analgesics. CNS Drugs 2013; 27:989.
49. GC McDowell 2nd and JE Pope. Intrathecal ziconotide: dosing and administration strategies in patients with refractory chronic pain. Neuromodulation 2016; 19:522.
50. Ziconotide (Prialt) for chronic pain. Med Lett Drugs Ther 2005; 47:103.
51. CJ Derry et al. Caffeine as an analgesic adjuvant for acute pain in adults. Cochrane Database Syst Rev 2014; 12:CD009281.
52. J Park and HJ Park. Botulinum toxin for the treatment of neuropathic pain. Toxins (Basel) 2017; 9:E260.
53. PF Whiting et al. Cannabinoids for medical use: a systematic review and meta-analysis. JAMA 2015; 313:2456.
54. Cannabis and cannabinoids. Med Lett Drugs Ther 2016; 58:97.
55. SM Nugent et al. The effects of cannabis among adults with chronic pain and an overview of general harms: a systematic review. Ann Intern Med 2017; 167:319.
56. PS Davies and BS Galer. Review of lidocaine patch 5% studies in the treatment of postherpetic neuralgia. Drugs 2004; 64:937.
57. Capsaicin patch (Qutenza) for postherpetic neuralgia. Med Lett Drugs Ther 2011; 53:42.

Nonopioid Drugs for Pain

58. FDA. Drug Safety Communication: rare cases of serious burns with the use of over-the-counter topical muscle and joint pain relievers. Available at www.fda.gov/Drugs/DrugSafety/ucm318858.htm. Accessed February 1, 2018.

59. J Schneiderhan et al. Primary care of patients with chronic pain. JAMA 2017; 317:2367.

60. RB Saper et al. Yoga, physical therapy, or education for chronic low back pain: a randomized noninferiority trial. Ann Intern Med 2017; 167:85.

61. LJ Geneen et al. Physical activity and exercise for chronic pain in adults: an overview of Cochrane Reviews. Cochrane Database Syst Rev 2017; 4:CD011279.

62. D Green et al. Effects of diflunisal on platelet function and fecal blood loss. Pharmacotherapy 1983; 3(2 pt 2):65S.

MANAGEMENT OF
Opioid Withdrawal Symptoms

Original publication date – August 2018

Pharmacologic management of opioid withdrawal symptoms can reduce the intensity of drug craving and improve treatment retention in patients with opioid use disorder who will receive maintenance treatment. Withdrawal management without subsequent maintenance treatment is associated with high rates of relapse, overdose death, and HIV and/or hepatitis C virus infection. Several guidelines on management of opioid withdrawal are available.[1-3] Maintenance treatment of opioid use disorder was reviewed in a previous issue.[4]

SYMPTOMS

Opioid withdrawal is not generally life-threatening. Symptoms such as nausea, vomiting, diarrhea, abdominal cramping, myalgia, increased lacrimation, mydriasis, piloerection, hyperhidrosis, agitation, and anxiety usually develop within 12 hours after the last use of a short-acting opioid (such as heroin or immediate-release hydrocodone) or within 30 hours after the last use of a long-acting opioid (such as methadone, extended-release oxycodone, or fentanyl transdermal patches).[5] They generally persist for about 3-5 days after discontinuation of a short-acting opioid or 10-14 days after stopping a longer-acting opioid, but can last longer in some patients. Withdrawal symptoms precipitated by administration of an opioid antagonist such as naloxone or naltrexone or a partial opioid agonist such as buprenorphine can be severe enough to require hospitalization.[6]

Recommendations
► Opioid withdrawal symptoms are generally managed with a slow taper of either the full opioid agonist methadone or the partial opioid agonist buprenorphine, with or without an alpha$_2$ adrenergic agonist.
► Buprenorphine with or without naloxone is the treatment of choice for most patients. It is comparable in efficacy to methadone, but it is safer and can be prescribed in an outpatient setting.
► Methadone is effective for management of symptoms, but its adverse effects and potential drug interactions are a concern, and it can only be administered in an inpatient setting or through a supervised treatment program. It should be used when buprenorphine is unavailable or ineffective, or in patients who would benefit from daily supervised dosing.
► The alpha$_2$ adrenergic agonists clonidine and lofexidine are less effective than methadone or buprenorphine. They are most useful as adjuncts to an opioid agonist and in settings where use of an opioid agonist is prohibited.
► Adjunctive treatment of specific withdrawal symptoms can improve patient comfort, and psychosocial therapy can improve rates of abstinence and treatment retention.
► Withdrawal management is not recommended in pregnant women, who should receive maintenance treatment with an opioid agonist.

BUPRENORPHINE

Buprenorphine is a mu-opioid receptor partial agonist and a kappa-opioid receptor antagonist. It is classified as a schedule III controlled substance (lower potential for abuse than schedule II; recognized medical use). Withdrawal management with buprenorphine can be performed in an outpatient setting; current laws relating to outpatient prescribing of buprenorphine are available on the website for the Substance Abuse and Mental Health Services Administration.[7]

Buprenorphine is available alone and in combination with the opioid antagonist naloxone.[8-10] Taken orally or sublingually, naloxone is poorly absorbed and generally has no clinical effects; combining buprenorphine with naloxone in sublingual or buccal formulations is intended to deter patients from modifying the dosage form for intranasal or parenteral administration.

EFFICACY — In a Cochrane review, buprenorphine and methadone were found to be similarly effective in reducing withdrawal symptoms. Buprenorphine was also found to be more effective than alpha$_2$ adrenergic agonists in relieving withdrawal symptoms and improving treatment retention.[11]

SAFETY — Buprenorphine is safer than methadone; it is a partial agonist and has a ceiling on its respiratory depressant effect. It also has a lower abuse potential than methadone; the abuse potential may be further reduced by the presence of naloxone in buprenorphine products.

In a retrospective analysis of adverse drug events reported to the FDA over 42 years, buprenorphine was significantly less likely than methadone to be associated with QT-interval prolongation, ventricular arrhythmia, or cardiac arrest.[12]

DRUG INTERACTIONS — Buprenorphine is metabolized primarily by CYP3A4; concomitant use with a CYP3A4 inducer can decrease serum concentrations of buprenorphine and use with a 3A4 inhibitor can increase them.[13] As with methadone or any other opioid, use of buprenorphine with selective serotonin reuptake inhibitors (SSRIs), serotonin and norepinephrine reuptake inhibitors (SNRIs), or other serotonergic drugs may result in serotonin syndrome, but many patients take these drugs together without adverse effects. Use of benzodiazepines or other sedating drugs with buprenorphine can result in additive effects. Buprenorphine has a greater affinity for opioid receptors than full opioid agonists such as heroin or morphine and can displace them, causing opioid withdrawal.

DOSAGE AND ADMINISTRATION — To prevent severe withdrawal symptoms, buprenorphine should not be started until the patient is already experiencing mild to moderate opioid withdrawal symptoms (Clinical Opiate Withdrawal Scale score ~11-12). The initial daily dose of 2-4 mg should be uptitrated as tolerated until a dose that

Table 1. Some Drugs for Management of Opioid Withdrawal Symptoms	
Drug	**Some Available Formulations**
Opioids	
Buprenorphine – generic	2, 8 mg sublingual tabs
Buprenorphine/naloxone –	
generic	2/0.5 mg, 8/2 mg sublingual tabs
Bunavail (Biodelivery Sciences)	2.1/0.3 mg, 4.2/0.7 mg, 6.3/1 mg buccal films
Suboxone (Indivior)	2/0.5 mg, 4/1 mg, 8/2 mg, 12/3 mg sublingual films
Zubsolv (Orexo)	1.4/0.36 mg, 2.9/0.71 mg, 5.7/1.4 mg, 8.6/2.1 mg, 11.4/2.9 mg sublingual tabs
Methadone – generic	5, 10 mg tabs; 5, 10 mg/5 mL oral solution; 10 mg/mL oral concentrate; 40 mg tabs for oral suspension[6]
Dolophine (Roxane)	5, 10 mg tabs[6]
Central Alpha₂ Adrenergic Agonists	
Clonidine[7] – generic	0.1, 0.2, 0.3 mg tabs
Catapres (Boehringer Ingelheim) transdermal weekly patch –	
generic	0.1, 0.2, 0.3 mg/24 hr patches
Catapres-TTS	
Lofexidine – *Lucemyra* (US WorldMeds/Salix)	0.18 mg tabs

1. Approximate WAC for 1 week's treatment at the lowest usual initial target dosage. WAC = wholesaler acquisition cost, or manufacturer's published price to wholesalers; WAC represents published catalogue or list prices and may not represent an actual transactional price. Source: AnalySource® Monthly. August 5, 2018. Reprinted with permission by First Databank, Inc. All rights reserved. ©2018. www.fdbhealth.com/policies/drug-pricing-policy.
2. To prevent severe withdrawal symptoms, treatment should not be started until the patient is experiencing mild to moderate symptoms (Clinical Opiate Withdrawal Scale score ~11-12).
3. The drug should be tapered in decrements of 10-20% every 1-2 days. Some patients, particularly those who are previously taking a long-acting opioid, may require a slower taper.
4. Some CYP rapid metabolizers may require more frequent dosing.
5. Cost of oral concentrate.
6. To reduce the risk of drug diversion, the liquid formulation, diluted in colored water or juice, is generally used in treatment programs.

suppresses withdrawal symptoms is reached (usually 8 mg/day, but some patients require up to 16 mg/day). The drug should then be tapered in decrements of 10-20% every 1-2 days. Some patients, particularly those who were previously taking a long-acting opioid, may require a slower taper.

Usual Initial Target Dosage	Cost[1]
8-16 mg once/d[2,3]	$23.10
8/2-16/4 mg once/d[2,3]	49.50
4.2/0.7-8.4/1.4 mg once/d[2,3]	54.30
8/2-16/4 mg once/d[2,3]	57.00
5.7/1.4-11.4/2.9 mg once/d[2,3]	58.10
20-30 mg once/d[3,4]	1.00[5]
	8.30
0.1-0.3 mg q6-8 hrs[8]	1.00
	52.80
See footnote 9	15.50[10]
	35.60[10]
0.54 mg qid[8,11]	1738.00

7. Not FDA-approved for this indication.
8. Can be used as the primary drug or as an adjunct to buprenorphine or methadone. The dose should be reduced, delayed, or withheld if clinically significant bradycardia and/or hypotension occur. After the period of peak withdrawal symptoms, the drug should be tapered by 0.1 mg (clonidine) or 0.18 mg (lofexidine) per dose every 1-2 days.
9. The clonidine patch should not be used initially because therapeutic serum clonidine concentrations are not achieved until 3 days after application.
10. Cost of one 0.3 mg/24 hr patch.
11. FDA-approved for up to 14 days' use. Doses should be taken 5-6 hours apart. Dosage can be increased to 0.72 mg qid if necessary. The maximum dosage in patients with a CrCl <90 and ≥30 mL/min or moderate hepatic impairment (Child-Pugh B) is 0.36 mg qid; in patients with a CrCl <30 mL/min or severe hepatic impairment (Child-Pugh C), it is 0.18 mg qid.

METHADONE

Methadone is a synthetic mu-opioid receptor agonist with a slow onset of action and a long, variable elimination half-life. At high doses, methadone induces cross-tolerance with other opioid agonists. Patients tolerant to other opioid agonists may have incomplete cross-tolerance to methadone.[14]

Methadone is classified as a schedule II controlled substance (highest potential for abuse; recognized medical use). By law, withdrawal management with methadone is restricted to an inpatient setting or a government-licensed opioid treatment program (OTP). The drug is available as oral tablets, tablets for oral suspension, an oral solution, and an oral concentrate. To reduce the risk of drug diversion, OTPs usually do not use the tablet formulation.[15]

EFFICACY — In a Cochrane review, methadone and buprenorphine were found to be similarly effective in reducing withdrawal symptoms.[11] In another review, treatment duration was significantly shorter with methadone than with alpha$_2$ adrenergic agonists.[16]

SAFETY — Methadone overdose can be fatal. The drug can accumulate during induction; it takes 4-7 days to reach steady state. In overdosage, or if the dose is increased too rapidly during initiation of therapy, methadone can cause sedation and respiratory depression. The respiratory depressant effect of methadone peaks later and lasts longer than that of buprenorphine and other opioid agonists.

Methadone can prolong the QT interval and cause arrhythmias such as torsades de pointes, particularly in patients taking other QT interval-prolonging drugs[17] and in those with congenital long QT syndrome or a history of QT-interval prolongation.

DRUG INTERACTIONS — Methadone is a substrate of CYP3A4, 2B6, 2C9, 2C19, and 2D6; inhibitors of one or more of these isozymes can increase serum concentrations of methadone, and inducers can reduce them.[13] Inhibition or induction of multiple isozymes increases the likelihood of a clinically significant interaction. Concurrent use of methadone and other QT interval-prolonging drugs should be avoided if possible.[17] As with any opioid, concomitant use of methadone with SSRIs, SNRIs, or other serotonergic drugs could result in serotonin syndrome, but many patients take these drugs together without adverse effects. Concurrent use of methadone and benzodiazepines or other sedating drugs can result in additive CNS effects.

DOSAGE AND ADMINISTRATION — The initial dosage of a methadone taper is usually 20-30 mg once daily; federal law prohibits administration of an initial methadone dose >30 mg or a total first daily dose >40 mg. The initial dose is then gradually tapered in decrements of 10-20% every 1-2 days. Some patients, particularly those who were previously taking a long-acting opioid, may require a slower taper.[18,19]

CLONIDINE

Clonidine is a centrally acting alpha$_2$ adrenergic agonist that has been used off-label to manage opioid withdrawal symptoms for more than 30 years. It is most effective at reducing the symptoms of opioid withdrawal related to noradrenergic overactivity, such as GI symptoms, hyperhidrosis, anxiety, and irritability. It can be used as the primary treatment or as an adjunct to buprenorphine or methadone. Clonidine is not a controlled substance, and there are no special restrictions on its use.

EFFICACY — In a Cochrane review, clonidine was found to be more effective than placebo in reducing the incidence of severe opioid withdrawal symptoms and increasing the probability of treatment completion. Treatment completion rates with clonidine were similar to those with methadone, but clonidine appears to be less effective than methadone in relieving withdrawal symptoms and more likely to cause adverse effects, such as hypotension.[16]

SAFETY — Dose-related hypotension, bradycardia, dry mouth, drowsiness, dizziness, constipation, and sedation occur commonly with use of clonidine.

Central alpha$_2$ adrenergic agonists can cause syncope; outpatients taking clonidine should be able to self-monitor for hypotension, orthostasis, and bradycardia. If such symptoms occur, the next dose of clonidine should be reduced, delayed, or skipped. Abrupt discontinuation of clonidine, however, can cause marked rebound hypertension.

DRUG INTERACTIONS — Use of other CNS depressants, such as alcohol, or hypotensive or bradycardic drugs, such as beta blockers, with clonidine can result in additive effects.

DOSAGE AND ADMINISTRATION — The usual dosage of clonidine for withdrawal management is 0.1-0.3 mg taken orally every 6-8 hours. Sedation or hypotension may be dose-limiting. After the period of peak withdrawal, the dosage of clonidine can be gradually reduced, generally by 0.1 mg per dose every 1 to 2 days.

Clonidine patches should not be used initially because therapeutic serum concentrations of the drug are not achieved until 3 days after application. Even after therapeutic levels are reached, use of the patches may be difficult because of the need for frequent dosage adjustment.

LOFEXIDINE

Lofexidine is also a centrally acting alpha$_2$ adrenergic agonist. It was approved by the FDA in 2018 for management of opioid withdrawal,[20] but has been available in Europe for this indication for more than 20 years. Like clonidine, lofexidine is not a controlled substance, and there are no special restrictions on its use, but it is much more expensive than clonidine.

EFFICACY — In two randomized, double-blind trials (one published; one summarized in the package insert) in a total of 866 adults who were physically dependent on short-acting opioids and were receiving inpatient treatment for withdrawal management, lofexidine significantly improved Subjective Opiate Withdrawal Scale (SOWS-Gossop) scores and treatment retention rates compared to placebo.[21] Direct comparisons between clonidine and lofexidine are limited; a Cochrane review found no difference in efficacy between the two drugs.[16]

SAFETY — Hypotension, orthostasis, bradycardia, dizziness, somnolence, sedation, dry mouth, and rebound blood pressure elevations occurred significantly more often with lofexidine than with placebo in clinical trials. Women were more likely than men to stop treatment because of bradycardia and orthostatic hypotension. Lofexidine appears to cause less hypotension than clonidine.[16]

Central alpha$_2$ adrenergic agonists can cause syncope; outpatients taking lofexidine should be able to self-monitor for hypotension, orthostasis, and bradycardia. If such symptoms occur, the next dose of lofexidine should be reduced, delayed, or skipped. Abrupt discontinuation of lofexidine, however, can cause marked rebound hypertension.

Lofexidine prolongs the QT interval. Electrolyte abnormalities should be corrected before treatment is started; ECG monitoring during treatment is recommended for patients with congestive heart failure, bradyarrhythmias, or hepatic or renal impairment. Lofexidine should not be used in patients with severe coronary insufficiency, recent myocardial infarction, congenital long QT syndrome, cerebrovascular disease, or marked bradycardia.

CYP2D6 poor metabolizers taking lofexidine may be at greater risk for adverse effects.

DRUG INTERACTIONS — Lofexidine should not be used concurrently with other drugs that cause bradycardia or hypotension. ECG monitoring during treatment is recommended for patients taking lofexidine concomitantly with other QT interval-prolonging drugs,[17] such as methadone. The strong CYP2D6 inhibitor paroxetine (*Paxil*, and others) increased lofexidine exposure by 28%; patients taking a CYP2D6 inhibitor[13] with lofexidine should be closely monitored for orthostatic hypotension and bradycardia.

DOSAGE AND ADMINISTRATION — Lofexidine is FDA-approved for up to 14 days' use. The recommended starting dosage is three 0.18-mg tablets taken four times daily, 5 to 6 hours apart. If necessary, the dosage can be increased to four tablets four times daily. After the period of peak withdrawal, the dosage of lofexidine can be gradually reduced, generally by one tablet per dose every 1 to 2 days. The maximum dosage of lofexidine in patients with a creatinine clearance (CrCl) <90 and ≥30 mL/min or moderate hepatic impairment (Child-Pugh B) is two tablets four times daily; in patients with a CrCl <30 mL/min or severe hepatic impairment (Child-Pugh C), it is one tablet four times daily.

ADJUNCTIVE TREATMENT

PHARMACOLOGIC — Adjunctive treatment is most likely to be needed in patients being treated primarily with an alpha$_2$ adrenergic agonist, but even those taking high doses of an opioid agonist may benefit from symptom-specific adjunctive pharmacotherapy.[22]

Anxiety and restlessness can be managed with a benzodiazepine such as lorazepam (but there is an increased risk of respiratory depression if the patient takes methadone or relapses) or a first-generation antihistamine such as hydroxyzine. **Diarrhea** can be treated with bismuth subsalicylate or the gut-specific opioid loperamide. **Abdominal cramping** can be managed with the antispasmodic dicyclomine. **Nausea and vomiting** can be treated with the 5-HT$_3$ receptor antagonist ondansetron (but not in patients taking methadone because of the risk of QT-interval prolongation) or a low dose of a phenothiazine such as prochlorperazine. **Insomnia** can be treated with a benzodiazepine receptor agonist such as zolpidem (also increases the risk of respiratory depression) or a low dose of a sedating antidepressant such as doxepin, trazodone, or mirtazapine. **Pain** should be managed with acetaminophen or a nonsteroidal anti-inflammatory drug (NSAID). **Muscle spasms** can be treated with a muscle relaxant such as cyclobenzaprine or baclofen.

NONPHARMACOLOGIC — Limited data suggest that combining pharmacologic withdrawal management with psychosocial therapies, such as psychotherapeutic counseling or provision of motivational incentives, can improve rates of abstinence and treatment retention and completion.[23]

ALTERNATIVE THERAPIES

Combining buprenorphine or an alpha$_2$ adrenergic agonist with low doses of the opioid antagonist **naltrexone** may shorten the duration of withdrawal management and allow for faster introduction of extended-release IM naltrexone, but it causes greater patient discomfort at the beginning of treatment.[24,25]

In **anesthesia-assisted (or ultra-rapid) opioid detoxification**, the patient is anesthetized, intubated, and mechanically ventilated, and then given a large dose of naloxone to precipitate acute withdrawal and a diuretic to accelerate renal clearance of the opioid. This practice has been associated with serious adverse events including cardiac arrest and death, and is not recommended.[26,27]

PREGNANCY

Opioid use during pregnancy is associated with an increased risk of complications such as preeclampsia, miscarriage, reduced fetal growth, fetal death, and premature delivery.[28] Pregnant women who are physically dependent on opioids should receive opioid agonist maintenance therapy with methadone or buprenorphine (without naloxone), which is safer than detoxification alone.[29] Infants born to mothers using opioids near delivery, including mothers taking buprenorphine or methadone, are at risk of neonatal opioid withdrawal.

LACTATION

Use of methadone or buprenorphine monotherapy by breastfeeding women is generally considered safe. Clonidine passes into human milk;

the labeling recommends caution when clonidine is administered to a breastfeeding woman. Lofexidine has not been studied in lactating women.

1. The American Society of Addiction Medicine. National practice guideline for the use of medications in the treatment of addiction involving opioid use. June 1, 2015. Available at: www.asam.org/docs/default-source/practice-support/guidelines-and-consensus-docs/asam-national-practice-guideline-supplement.pdf. Accessed August 9, 2018.
2. MA Schuckit. Treatment of opioid-use disorders. N Engl J Med 2016; 375:357.
3. British Columbia Ministry of Health. A guideline for the clinical management of opioid use disorder. June 5, 2017. Available at: https://www2.gov.bc.ca/assets/gov/health/practitioner-pro/bc-guidelines/opioid-use-disorder.pdf.
4. Drugs for opioid use disorder. Med Lett Drugs Ther 2017; 59:89.
5. Opioids for pain. Med Lett Drugs Ther 2018; 60:57.
6. H Hassanian-Moghaddam et al. Withdrawal syndrome caused by naltrexone in opioid abusers. Hum Exp Toxicol 2014; 33:561.
7. Substance Abuse and Mental Health Services Administration. Buprenorphine waiver management. January 18, 2018. Available at: www.samhsa.gov/programs-campaigns/medication-assisted-treatment/training-materials-resources/buprenorphine-waiver. Accessed August 9, 2018.
8. Buprenorphine: an alternative to methadone. Med Lett Drugs Ther 2003; 45:13.
9. In brief: Buprenorphine/naloxone (Zubsolv) for opioid dependence. Med Lett Drugs Ther 2013; 55:83.
10. Bunavail: another buprenorphine/naloxone formulation for opioid dependence. Med Lett Drugs Ther 2015; 57:19.
11. L Gowing et al. Buprenorphine for managing opioid withdrawal. Cochrane Database Syst Rev 2017; 2:CD002025.
12. DP Kao et al. Arrhythmia associated with buprenorphine and methadone reported to the Food and Drug Administration. Addiction 2015; 110:1468.
13. Inhibitors and inducers of CYP enzymes and P-glycoprotein. Med Lett Drugs Ther 2017 September 18 (epub). Available at: www.medicalletter.org/downloads/CYP_PGP_Tables.pdf. Accessed August 9, 2018.
14. Institute for Safe Medication Practices. Keeping patients safe from iatrogenic methadone overdoses. February 14, 2008. Available at: www.ismp.org/resources/keeping-patients-safe-iatrogenic-methadone-overdoses. Accessed August 9, 2018.
15. Substance Abuse and Mental Health Services Administration. Emerging issues in the use of methadone. Substance abuse treatment advisory: news for the treatment field. Spring 2009; 8:1. Available at: https://store.samhsa.gov/shin/content/SMA09-4368/SMA09-4368.pdf. Accessed August 9, 2018.
16. L Gowing et al. Alpha₂-adrenergic agonists for the management of opioid withdrawal. Cochrane Database Syst Rev 2016; 5:CD002024.
17. RL Woosley and KA Romero. QT drugs list. Available at: www.crediblemeds.org. Accessed August 9, 2018.
18. NM Wright et al. Comparison of methadone and buprenorphine for opiate detoxification (LEEDS trial): a randomised controlled trial. Br J Gen Pract 2011; 61:e772.

19. U.S. Government Publishing Office. 42 CFR 8.12 – Federal opioid treatment standards. Available at: www.gpo.gov/fdsys/pkg/CFR-2017-title42-vol1/pdf/CFR-2017-title42-vol1-sec8-12.pdf. Accessed August 9, 2018.

20. Lofexidine (Lucemyra) for opioid withdrawal. Med Lett Drugs Ther 2018; 60:115.

21. CW Gorodetzky et al. A phase III, randomized, multi-center, double blind, placebo controlled study of safety and efficacy of lofexidine for relief of symptoms in individuals undergoing inpatient opioid withdrawal. Drug Alcohol Depend 2017; 176:79.

22. W Ling et al. A multi-center randomized trial of buprenorphine-naloxone versus clonidine for opioid detoxification: findings from the National Institute on Drug Abuse Clinical Trials Network. Addiction 2005; 100:1090.

23. L Amato et al. Psychosocial and pharmacological treatments versus pharmacological treatments for opioid detoxification. Cochrane Database Syst Rev 2011; 9:CD005031.

24. L Gowing et al. Opioid antagonists with minimal sedation for opioid withdrawal. Cochrane Database Syst Rev 2017; 5:CD002021.

25. American Society of Addiction Medicine. Public policy statement on rapid and ultra rapid opioid detoxification. 2005. Available at: www.asam.org/docs/default-source/public-policy-statements/1rod-urod---rev-of-oadusa-4-051.pdf. Accessed August 9, 2018.

26. SC Sigmon et al. Opioid detoxification and naltrexone induction strategies: recommendations for clinical practice. Am J Drug Alcohol Abuse 2012; 38:187.

27. CDC. Deaths and severe adverse events associated with anesthesia-assisted rapid opioid detoxification – New York City, 2012. MMWR Morb Mortal Wkly Rep 2013; 62:777.

28. ACOG Committee on Health Care for Underserved Women and American Society of Addiction Medicine. ACOG committee opinion No. 524: opioid abuse, dependence, and addiction in pregnancy. Obstet Gynecol 2012; 119:1070.

29. KA Saia et al. Caring for pregnant women with opioid use disorder in the USA: expanding and improving treatment. Curr Obstet Gynecol Rep 2016; 5:257.

Opioids for Pain

Original publication date – April 2018 (revised May 2018)

For use of nonopioid drugs for pain, see pages 129-152.[1]

ACUTE PAIN — For many types of moderate to severe acute pain, acetaminophen and/or an NSAID may be as effective as an opioid.[2] Short-acting formulations of full opioid agonists should generally be used for acute pain that is severe enough to require treatment with an opioid. Use of extended-release or long-acting opioid formulations initially and treatment durations >1 week have been associated with an increased risk of unintended long-term use.[3,4]

CHRONIC PAIN — Full opioid agonists are used for treatment of severe chronic cancer pain. Use of opioids for treatment of chronic noncancer pain is controversial; evidence of long-term effectiveness from controlled trials is limited and serious adverse effects such as overdose or opioid use disorder can occur.[5,6] Nonpharmacologic therapy and nonopioid pharmacologic therapy are preferred and may be as effective as an opioid for many types of chronic pain.[7] New US guidelines on prescribing opioids for chronic noncancer pain have been published (see Table 1).[8,9]

DOSAGE — Opioid dosage requirements vary widely from one patient to another. In general, experts recommend starting with the lowest available

---

Recommendations for Treatment of Pain

Acute Pain

► For **mild to moderate acute pain**, nonopioid analgesics such as aspirin, acetaminophen, or NSAIDs are preferred.

► For **localized pain**, topical agents, such as topical diclofenac or lidocaine, can be used alone or as adjunctive treatment.

► For **severe acute pain,** short-acting formulations of full opioid agonists may be necessary; they should be used at the lowest effective dose for the shortest time possible (usually ≤7 days).

Chronic Noncancer Pain

► Nonpharmacologic therapy and nonopioid pharmacologic therapy are preferred for treatment of chronic noncancer pain.

► For severe chronic noncancer pain that has not responded to other treatments, use of opioids may be necessary.

Chronic Cancer Pain

► Full opioid agonists are generally the drugs of choice for severe chronic cancer pain.

► Unlike NSAIDs, morphine and the other full opioid agonists generally have no dose ceiling for their analgesic effectiveness except that imposed by adverse effects.

► Patients who do not respond to one opioid may respond to another.

► Tolerance to most of the adverse effects of opioids, except constipation, develops at least as rapidly as tolerance to the analgesic effect; tolerance can usually be surmounted and adequate analgesia restored by increasing the dose or switching to another opioid.

► When frequent dosing becomes impractical, extended-release or long-acting opioids may be helpful.

Neuropathic Pain

► For initial treatment of neuropathic pain, an antidepressant or an antiepileptic can be used; combining them may produce a synergistic analgesic effect.

► For localized neuropathic pain, topical agents such as lidocaine and capsaicin can be used.

► For severe pain that has not responded to other agents, use of opioids may be necessary.

---

strength of a short-acting opioid and titrating to effect; a reasonable starting dose is 10 mg of oral morphine per 70 kg of body weight, or its equivalent (see MME conversion factors in Table 2). The lowest dose that maintains optimum pain relief with tolerable side effects should be used; high doses have been associated with a higher incidence of overdose deaths.[10] After initial titration with a short-acting formulation and determination of the 24-hour dose requirement, an extended-release or long-acting formulation can be used in patients requiring around-the-clock dosing. In palliative care and active cancer pain treatment, rapid-onset opioids should be available for breakthrough pain.

ADVERSE EFFECTS — Sedation, dizziness, nausea, vomiting, pruritus, sweating, and constipation are the most common adverse effects of opioids; respiratory depression is the most serious. Taken in usual doses, opioids, including mixed agonist/antagonists, may decrease respiratory drive and cause apnea in opioid-naive patients, particularly those who have chronic obstructive pulmonary disease, cor pulmonale, decreased respiratory reserve, or pre-existing respiratory depression. Tolerance to the respiratory depressant effect develops with chronic use.

Administration of naloxone can reverse severe respiratory depression resulting from an opioid overdose. Naloxone has a short half-life and repeated dosing may be needed, especially for overdose with a long-acting or extended-release opioid agonist.

Persistent opioid-induced sedation that limits activity can be ameliorated by giving small oral doses of stimulants such as methylphenidate (*Ritalin*, and others) in the morning and early afternoon. Modafinil (*Provigil*, and generics) has been shown (off label) to be beneficial in patients with opioid-induced sedation.[11]

Tolerance usually develops rapidly to the sedative and emetic effects of opioids, but not to constipation; a stimulant or osmotic laxative with or without a stool softener should be started early in treatment. Three peripherally-acting mu-opioid receptor antagonists, methylnaltrexone *(Relistor)*, naloxegol *(Movantik)*, and naldemedine *(Symproic)*, are FDA-approved for treatment of opioid-induced constipation. They appear to be similar in efficacy and safety, but no direct comparisons are available.[12-14] Lubiprostone *(Amitiza)*, an oral chloride channel activator, appears to be less effective. Transdermal fentanyl may cause less constipation than sustained-release oral morphine.[15]

Opioid-induced hyperalgesia has been reported in some patients treated with high doses of opioids. These patients experience worsening pain that cannot be overcome simply by increasing the dose (as is the case in tolerance), but rather only by reducing the dose, completely discontinuing the opioid, or switching to another opioid.[16]

Chronic use of opioids can increase prolactin levels and reduce levels of sex hormones, resulting in reduced sexual function, decreased libido, infertility, mood disturbances, and bone loss.[17] Cases of adrenal insufficiency have been reported, particularly after >1 month of opioid use.[18]

TOLERANCE — Tolerance develops with chronic use of opioids; the patient first notices a reduction in adverse effects and a shorter duration of analgesia, followed by a decrease in the effectiveness of each dose. Tolerance to most of the adverse effects of opioids (except constipation) develops at least as rapidly as tolerance to the analgesic effect; it can usually be surmounted and adequate analgesia restored by increasing the dose or switching to a different opioid. Cross-tolerance exists among all full agonists, but is not complete; when switching to another opioid, reducing the calculated equianalgesic dose by at least 25-50% is recommended (see MME conversion factors in Table 2). Switching opioid-tolerant patients to methadone may improve pain relief, but should be done cautiously; the equianalgesic dose of methadone is not well-established in opioid-tolerant patients.

PHYSICAL DEPENDENCE — Clinically significant dependence can develop after several days to weeks of continued treatment with an opioid. Withdrawal symptoms will occur if the drug is discontinued suddenly or

Table 1. Opioid Prescribing for Chronic Noncancer Pain[1,2]
► Nonpharmacologic therapy and nonopioid pharmacologic therapy are preferred. Opioid therapy should be considered only if expected benefits for pain and function are anticipated to outweigh risks to the patient.
► Before starting opioid therapy, treatment goals for pain and function should be established.
► Opioid treatment of chronic noncancer pain (duration >3 months) should be combined with nonpharmacologic therapy and nonopioid pharmacologic therapy.
► Short-acting opioids are recommended for initial treatment; the lowest effective dose should be used.
► Extended-release or long-acting opioids should be reserved for patients with severe, continuous pain who have received short-acting opioids daily for >1 week.
► Benefits and risks should be evaluated within 1-4 weeks of starting treatment or of dose escalation, and at least every 3 months with continued treatment.
► Higher opioid doses are associated with increased risks for motor vehicle injury, opioid use disorder, and overdose. Risk/benefit should be reassessed before increasing dosage to >50 oral morphine milligram equivalents (MMEs)/day. Dosages >90 MMEs/day should be avoided if possible.
► If pain relief is inadequate, opioid therapy is poorly tolerated, or there is evidence of misuse, other treatments should be optimized and opioids should be tapered to a lower dosage or tapered and discontinued.
► The opioid antagonist naloxone should be offered to patients at risk of opioid overdose.
► State prescription drug monitoring program data can be used to determine whether a patient is receiving opioid dosages or combination treatments that increase the risk for overdose.
► Urine drug testing is recommended before starting treatment and at least annually thereafter to assess for use of other controlled prescription drugs and/or illicit drugs.
► Medication-assisted treatment should be arranged for patients who develop opioid use disorder.
1. D Dowell et al. MMWR Recomm Rep 2016; 65:1. 2. L Manchikanti et al. Pain Physician 2017; 20 (2S):S3.

an opioid antagonist or partial agonist is given. Opioids should be tapered to reduce withdrawal symptoms.

DRUG INTERACTIONS — Use of opioids with alcohol, general anesthetics, phenothiazines, sedative-hypnotics such as benzodiazepines or barbiturates, tricyclic antidepressants, or other CNS depressants increases the risk of respiratory depression and death.[19] Urinary retention and severe constipation, possibly leading to paralytic ileus, could occur with concurrent use of an opioid and an anticholinergic drug. Use of opioids with serotonergic drugs has resulted in serotonin syndrome; cases have been reported more frequently with fentanyl, meperidine, methadone, tapentadol, and tramadol.[18] Use of an opioid with or within 14 days of an MAO inhibitor may result in serotonin syndrome or opioid toxicity and is not recommended.

Buprenorphine, fentanyl, hydrocodone, meperidine, methadone, oxycodone, and tramadol are metabolized by CYP3A4. Concurrent administration of a drug that inhibits CYP3A4 (or discontinuation of a CYP3A4 inducer) can increase serum concentrations of these drugs and the risk of sedation and respiratory depression. Concurrent use of a drug that induces CYP3A4 (or discontinuation of a CYP3A4 inhibitor) could decrease their serum concentrations and analgesic effect, possibly leading to withdrawal symptoms. Concomitant use of methadone with CYP2B6, 2C19, 2C9, or 2D6 inhibitors (or discontinuation of inducers of these enzymes) may increase methadone plasma concentrations.[20]

Patients taking codeine or tramadol who are concurrently taking drugs that inhibit CYP2D6 may not experience an analgesic effect.

Concomitant use with cimetidine could potentiate the effects of morphine. Coadministration of P-glycoprotein inhibitors such as amiodarone can increase morphine exposure by about two-fold.[20]

PREGNANCY — Opioid use during pregnancy has been associated with preterm delivery, poor fetal growth, stillbirth, and birth defects, including neural tube defects, congenital heart defects, and gastroschisis.[21] It can also lead to neonatal opioid withdrawal syndrome. Opioid withdrawal during pregnancy has been associated with spontaneous abortion and premature labor. Pregnant women who are physically dependent on opioids should receive opioid agonist maintenance therapy with buprenorphine or methadone. Neonatal toxicity and death have been reported in breastfed infants whose mothers were taking codeine.[8]

FULL OPIOID AGONISTS

CODEINE — Codeine is an oral opioid agonist with a long history of use as an analgesic and cough suppressant. It is a prodrug that is converted to morphine by CYP2D6. Patients who are CYP2D6 poor metabolizers (up to 10% of the population) or are taking drugs that inhibit CYP2D6, such as fluoxetine, may not be able to convert codeine to morphine and may not experience an analgesic effect. Patients who are CYP2D6 ultra-rapid metabolizers rapidly convert codeine to higher-than-usual levels of morphine, which may result in toxicity.

The FDA has issued warnings about the use of codeine in children due to concerns about the risk of respiratory depression and death. It is contraindicated for use in children <12 years old and in those <18 years old following tonsillectomy or adenoidectomy. It should be avoided in children 12-18 years old who are obese or have an increased risk of serious breathing problems and in breastfeeding women.[22]

FENTANYL — Fentanyl is available in parenteral, transdermal, intranasal, and oral transmucosal formulations. It is FDA-approved only for use in opioid-tolerant patients. Fentanyl should be started only after initial titration with a short-acting opioid.

Patients should be warned that exposing a fentanyl patch to heat from an external source (e.g., a heating pad), increased exertion, or high fever could increase release of the drug and the risk of respiratory depression.[23] Deaths have occurred in children following accidental exposure to the patch. The FDA recommends disposing of the patch by folding the sticky sides together and flushing it down the toilet.[24]

Table 2. Some Oral/Topical Opioid Analgesics

Drug	Some Oral/Topical Formulations
Full Agonists	
Codeine – generic	15, 30, 60 mg tabs
Fentanyl	
transdermal – generic	12, 25, 37.5, 50, 62.5, 75, 87.5, 100 mcg/hr patches
Duragesic (Janssen)	12, 25, 50, 75, 100 mcg/hr patches
transmucosal –	
Abstral (Sentynl)	100, 200, 300, 400, 600, 800 mcg sublingual tabs
Actiq (Teva)	200, 400, 600, 800, 1200, 1600 mcg transmucosal
generic	lozenges
Fentora (Cephalon)	100, 200, 400, 600, 800 mcg buccal tabs
Lazanda (Depomed)	100, 300, 400 mcg/100 mcL nasal spray
Subsys (Insys)	100, 200, 400, 600, 800, 1200, 1600 mcg sublingual spray

*FDA-approved as an abuse-deterrent formulation; ER = extended-release; MME = oral morphine milligram equivalent; N.A. = price not yet available

1. Dosage adjustment for renal or hepatic impairment may be necessary.
2. Dosage for patients who are opioid-naive or opioid-nontolerant (except for products such as fentanyl that are not recommended for such patients).
2a. In general, experts recommend starting with the lowest available strength of a short-acting opioid and titrating to effect; a reasonable starting dose is 10 mg of morphine per 70 kg of body weight, or its equivalent (see MME conversion factors in footnote 5).
3 Approximate WAC for 30 days' treatment at the lowest usual adult oral starting dosage or with the lowest available strength. WAC = wholesaler acquisition cost or manufacturer's published price to wholesalers; WAC represents a published catalogue or list price and may not represent an actual transactional price. Source: AnalySource® Monthly. March 5, 2018. Reprinted with permission by First Databank, Inc. All rights reserved. ©2018. www.fdbhealth.com/policies/drug-pricing-policy.
4. Single-agent codeine is schedule II; fixed-dose combinations containing acetaminophen are schedule III or V.

Usual Adult Oral Starting Dosage[1,2,2a]	Comments	Cost[3]
15-60 mg q4h	▶ Schedule II-V[4] controlled substance ▶ MME conversion factor[5]: 0.15 ▶ Also available parenterally ▶ Also available in fixed-dose combinations with acetaminophen ▶ Contraindicated in children <12 years old and all children post-adenotonsillectomy	$66.40

See footnotes 8,9	▶ Schedule II controlled substance
	▶ MME conversion factor[5]: patch[6]: 2.4
	  tabs/lozenges[7]: 0.13
	  sublingual spray[7]: 0.18
	  nasal spray[7]: 0.16
		162.40
		357.50

100 mcg 200 mcg	▶ Also available parenterally ▶ Not recommended for opioid-naive patients	43.70[10] 57.30[10] 12.20[10]
100 mcg 100 mcg 100 mcg	▶ Abstral, Actiq, Fentora, Lazanda, and Subsys are indicated only for breakthrough pain in opioid-tolerant patients with cancer ▶ Actiq may cause dental caries	49.20[10] 108.20[10] 58.90[10]

5. To convert the total daily dose of an opioid (except fentanyl: see footnotes 6 and 7) to MMEs, multiply its dose in mg/day by the conversion factor. The conversion factor is an estimate and should not be used to determine the dosage for converting patients from one opioid to another. When converting patients from one opioid to another, the new opioid is typically dosed substantially lower (25-50%) than the calculated dose in MMEs (CDC National Center for Injury Prevention and Control. Available at: www.cdc.gov/drugoverdose/resources/data.html).
6. To convert the fentanyl patch to the MME dose/day, multiply the dose in mcg/h by the conversion factor.
7. To convert fentanyl transmucosal products to MMEs, multiply the number of micrograms in a given unit by the conversion factor.
8. Starting dose determined by previous opioid dosage. Extended-release/long-acting formulations are generally not recommended for opioid-naive patients.
9. Not recommended for opioid-nontolerant patients. The recommended dosing interval is 72 hours. Some patients need to change the patch every 48 hours to achieve adequate analgesia.
10. Cost for a single lozenge, tablet, or spray of the lowest available strength.

Continued on next page

Opioids for Pain

Table 2. Some Oral/Topical Opioid Analgesics (continued)

Drug	Some Oral/Topical Formulations
Hydrocodone – extended-release *Hysingla ER* (Purdue)* *Zohydro ER* (Pernix)	20, 30, 40, 60, 80, 100, 120 mg ER tabs 10, 15, 20, 30, 40, 50 mg ER caps
Benzhydrocodone/ acetaminophen – *Apadaz* (Kempharm)	6.12 mg/325 mg tabs
Hydromorphone – generic *Dilaudid* (Rhodes) extended-release – generic *Exalgo* (Mallinckrodt)	2, 4, 8 mg tabs; 5 mg/5 mL PO soln 8, 12, 16, 32 mg ER tabs
Levorphanol – generic	2 mg tabs
Meperidine – generic *Demerol* (Validus)	50, 100 mg tabs; 50 mg/5 mL PO soln 100 mg tabs

*FDA-approved as an abuse-deterrent formulation; ER = extended-release; MME = oral morphine milligram equivalent; N.A. = price not yet available

Usual Adult Oral Starting Dosage[1,2,2a]	Comments	Cost[3]
20 mg q24h[8] 10 mg q12h[8]	► Schedule II controlled substance ► MME conversion factor[5]: 1 ► Immediate-release formulations only available in fixed-dose combinations with acetaminophen (*Vicodin*, *Norco*, others) or ibuprofen (*Vicoprofen*, others)	$258.80 514.20
6.12 mg/325 mg q4-6h	► Schedule II controlled substance ► Prodrug of hydrocodone ► Only available in a fixed-dose combination with acetaminophen	N.A.
2 mg q6-8h See footnote 8	► Schedule II controlled substance ► MME conversion factor[5]: 4 ► Also available in parenteral formulations, including a high-potency injectable (*Dilaudid HP*, generics), and as a suppository	13.70 179.60 292.50[11] 418.40[11]
2 mg q6-8h	► Schedule II controlled substance ► MME conversion factor[5]: 11 ► Accumulation may occur with chronic use	3690.00
50 mg q3-4h	► Schedule II controlled substance ► MME conversion factor[5]: 0.1 ► Also available parenterally ► More rapid onset of action than morphine ► Tissue irritation occurs with parenteral use ► Use should be limited to ≤48 hours	8.90[12] 26.10[12]

11. Cost of 30 8-mg tablets.
12. Cost for 2 days' treatment.

Continued on next page

Table 2. Some Oral/Topical Opioid Analgesics (continued)

Drug	Some Oral/Topical Formulations
Methadone – generic	5, 10 mg tabs; 5, 10 mg/5 mL PO soln; 10 mg/mL PO conc; 40 mg tabs for PO susp
Dolophine (West-Ward)	5, 10 mg tabs
Morphine – generic extended-release –	15, 30 mg tabs; 10, 20, 100 mg/5 mL PO soln
Arymo ER (Egalet)*	15, 30, 60 mg ER tabs
MS Contin (Rhodes) generic	15, 30, 60, 100, 200 mg ER tabs
Kadian (Actavis)	10, 20, 30, 40, 50, 60, 70, 80, 100, 200 mg ER caps
generic	10, 20, 30, 50, 60, 80, 100 mg ER caps
multiphase generic[15]	30, 45, 60, 75, 90, 120 mg ER caps
Morphabond ER (Sankyo)*	15, 30, 60, 100 mg ER tabs
Morphine/naltrexone – extended-release –	
Embeda (Pfizer)*	20/0.8, 30/1.2, 50/2, 60/2.4, 80/3.2, 100/4 mg ER caps

*FDA-approved as an abuse-deterrent formulation; ER = extended-release; MME = oral morphine milligram equivalent; N.A. = price not yet available
13. The methadone conversion factor increases at higher doses.

Usual Adult Oral Starting Dosage[1,2,2a]	Comments	Cost[3]
2.5-10 mg q8-12h[8]	► Schedule II controlled substance	$8.90
	► MME conversion factor[5,13]:	
	1-20 mg/d: 4	10.90
	21-40 mg/d: 8	
	41-60 mg/d: 10	
	61-80 mg/d:12	
	► Also available parenterally	
	► Accumulation may occur with chronic use	
10-30 mg q4h	► Schedule II controlled substance	39.90[14]
	► Also available for parenteral use and as	
15 mg q8 or 12h[8]	a suppository	284.90
15-30 mg q8-12h[8]	► Taking *Kadian* or multiphase ER caps	216.60
	with alcohol can result in rapid release	68.70
30 mg q24h[8]	of morphine	349.10
	► Maximum dose of multiphase ER caps	136.50
30 mg q24h[8]	is 1600 mg due to renal toxicity of	137.50
15 mg q12h[8]	fumaric acid in the beads (chewing or	324.00
	crushing the beads can be fatal)	
	► Schedule II controlled substance	
	► Naltrexone is only absorbed if the cap-	
20 mg/0.8 mg q24h[8]	sules are crushed, chewed, or dissolved	200.50
	► Taking *Embeda* with alcohol can result	
	in increased plasma levels of morphine	

14. Cost of 15-mg tabs.
15. Generic equivalent of *Avinza*, which has been discontinued.

Continued on next page

Table 2. Some Oral/Topical Opioid Analgesics (continued)

Drug	Some Oral/Topical Formulations
Oxycodone – generic	5 mg caps; 5, 10, 15, 20, 30 mg tabs; 5, 100 mg/5 mL PO soln
Oxaydo (Egalet)	5, 7.5 mg tabs
Roxybond (Daiichi Sankyo)*	5, 15, 30 mg tabs
extended-release –	
OxyContin (Purdue)* generic	10, 15, 20, 30, 40, 60, 80 mg ER tabs
Xtampza ER (Collegium)*	9, 13.5, 18, 27, 36 mg ER caps
Oxymorphone – generic	5, 10 mg tabs
Opana (Endo)	
extended-release – generic	5, 7.5, 10, 15, 20, 30, 40 mg ER tabs
Full Agonist/Reuptake Inhibitors	
Tapentadol –	
Nucynta (Collegium)	50, 75, 100 mg tabs
extended-release –	
Nucynta ER	50, 100, 150, 200, 250 mg ER tabs
Tramadol – generic	50 mg tabs
Ultram (Janssen)	
extended-release –	
generic[16]	100, 200, 300 mg ER tabs
multiphase generic[17]	100, 200, 300 mg ER tabs
ConZip (Vertical)	100, 200, 300 mg ER caps[18]
biphasic generic	100, 150, 200, 300 mg ER caps[18]

*FDA-approved as an abuse-deterrent formulation; ER = extended-release; MME = oral morphine milligram equivalent; N.A. = price not yet available
16. Generic equivalent of Ultram ER, which has been discontinued.
17. Generic equivalent of Ryzolt, which has been discontinued.

Usual Adult Oral Starting Dosage[1,2,2a]	Comments	Cost[3]
5-15 mg q4-6h	▸ Schedule II controlled substance	$14.90
5-15 mg q4-6h	▸ MME conversion factor[5]: 1.5	801.80
5-15 mg q4-6h	▸ Also available in fixed-dose combinations with acetaminophen (*Percocet*, others), aspirin (*Percodan*, others), or ibuprofen (*Combunox*, others)	800.40
10 mg q12h[8]		220.50
		226.40
9 mg q12h[8]		243.30
5-15 mg q4-6h	▸ Schedule II controlled substance	121.20
	▸ MME conversion factor[5]: 3	825.90
5 mg q12h[8]	▸ Also available parenterally	119.20
50-100 mg q4-6h	▸ Schedule II controlled substance	
	▸ MME conversion factor[5]: 0.4	694.60
	▸ Fewer GI adverse effects, but similar CNS effects compared to some other	
50 mg bid[8]	opioid agonists	374.00
50-100 mg q4-6h	▸ Schedule IV controlled substance	5.60
	▸ MME conversion factor[5]: 0.1	385.70
	▸ 50 mg equivalent to codeine 60 mg;	
100 mg once/d[8]	100 mg comparable to aspirin 650 mg	57.00
100 mg once/d[8]	plus codeine 60 mg	20.00
100 mg once/d[8]	▸ Also available in fixed-dose combinations with acetaminophen (*Ultracet*, others)	287.70
100 mg once/d[8]		229.60
	▸ Contraindicated in children <12 years old and all children post-adenotonsillectomy	
	▸ Starting with 25 mg/day and slowly titrating to usual dose over a few weeks may improve tolerability	
	▸ Maximum dose is 400 mg/d for short-acting formulations and 300 mg/d for ER formulations	

18. Mixture of immediate-release (IR) and extended-release (ER) tramadol: 100 mg contains 25 mg IR and 75 mg ER, 150 mg contains 37.5 mg IR and 112.5 mg ER, 200 mg contains 50 mg IR and 150 mg ER, 300 mg contains 50 mg IR and 250 mg ER.

HYDROCODONE — Hydrocodone is a semi-synthetic opioid that is partly metabolized by CYP2D6 to hydromorphone after oral administration. Short-acting formulations have been available for many years in combination with acetaminophen or ibuprofen. These combinations are the most abused opioids in the US. Extended-release, single-entity, oral formulations of hydrocodone *(Zohydro ER, Hysingla ER)* are available for management of severe pain; they permit higher dosing than the short-acting combination formulations.[25,26]

Coadministration of 40% alcohol with *Zohydro ER* resulted in a 2.4-fold increase in peak concentrations of hydrocodone; patients taking *Zohydro ER* should not consume alcoholic beverages or other products that contain alcohol.

The FDA has approved an oral, short-acting, fixed-dose combination of **benzhydrocodone**, a prodrug of hydrocodone, and acetaminophen *(Apadaz)* for short-term (<14 days) management of acute pain severe enough to require an opioid analgesic and for which alternative treatment options are inadequate. The combination is available as tablets containing benzhydrocodone 6.12 mg/acetaminophen 325 mg that are equivalent to short-acting hydrocodone 7.5 mg/acetaminophen 325 mg formulations. Abuse-deterrence studies were done, but did not show that the new combination is less likely to be abused by the oral or intranasal route than hydrocodone/acetaminophen combinations.

HYDROMORPHONE — A semi-synthetic opioid and a metabolite of hydrocodone, hydromorphone is available in parenteral, rectal, and short-acting and extended-release oral formulations.[27] In an open-label study in patients with chronic noncancer pain, once-daily hydromorphone was similar in efficacy to twice-daily oxycodone and caused less somnolence.[28] Starting dosages should be reduced in patients with moderate to severe renal impairment.

LEVORPHANOL — Oral levorphanol is used to treat chronic pain. It has a long half-life (16-18 hours) and can accumulate with repeated dosing.

Levorphanol exhibits incomplete cross-tolerance when converting from other opioids and requires careful dose titration.

MEPERIDINE — Meperidine should only be used for short-term (24-48 hours) treatment of moderate to severe acute pain. It has a more rapid onset of action than morphine, but is shorter acting. Meperidine has poor oral bioavailability, is highly irritating to tissues when given subcutaneously, and can cause muscle fibrosis when given intramuscularly.

Repeated doses of meperidine can lead to accumulation of normeperidine, a toxic metabolite with a 15- to 30-hour half-life. Normeperidine can cause dysphoria, irritability, tremor, myoclonus, and, occasionally, seizures, particularly with postoperative patient-controlled analgesia, or in elderly patients or those with impaired renal function.

In patients who are taking or have recently stopped taking an MAO inhibitor, use of meperidine can cause severe encephalopathy and death.

METHADONE — Methadone is available parenterally and orally for treatment of chronic pain, and orally for maintenance treatment of opioid use disorder. In one study, methadone was similar in efficacy to long-acting morphine for first-line treatment of cancer pain.[29] The plasma half-life of methadone is variable (can be as long as 5 days) and does not correlate with the duration of analgesia; close monitoring is required during the titration period because repeated doses can lead to accumulation, CNS depression, and death. In comparison to other opioids, use of methadone for pain relief has been associated with a higher risk of death from overdose.[30]

In addition to being a mu-agonist, methadone is also an NMDA (N-methyl-D-aspartate) receptor antagonist. NMDA receptor antagonism can be helpful when patients do not respond to other opioids, particularly when the pain has a neuropathic component. Methadone is not fully cross-tolerant with other opioid agonists. Switching from another opioid agonist to methadone should be done cautiously; the equianalgesic dose of methadone is not well established in opioid-tolerant patients.

Methadone has no active metabolites, which may be advantageous in patients with renal impairment. Dose-related QT interval prolongation, torsades de pointes, and death have been reported.[31]

MORPHINE — Morphine is available orally and parenterally. Given orally, morphine is well absorbed but undergoes extensive first-pass metabolism, resulting in a bioavailability of about 35%. Morphine should be used with caution in patients with severe renal impairment because accumulation of its metabolites can occur; increased concentrations of morphine-3-glucuronide, a neurotoxic metabolite, may cause agitation, confusion, delirium, and other adverse effects.

OXYCODONE — Oxycodone, a semi-synthetic opioid, is only available orally in the US. It is frequently used in combination with acetaminophen for treatment of acute pain. A long-acting formulation is commonly used for treatment of chronic cancer pain.

OXYMORPHONE — A metabolite of oxycodone, oxymorphone is available in parenteral and in short-acting and extended-release oral formulations.[32] *Opana ER,* an oral extended-release formulation of oxymorphone, has been removed from the market due to a high risk of serious adverse events when abused by injection; generic formulations of oral extended-release oxymorphone remain in production.

ABUSE-DETERRENT OPIOIDS — Several full-agonist opioids are available in abuse-deterrent formulations, both alone and in combination with opioid antagonists; there are no generic equivalents to these products (see Table 2). These formulations have one or more properties that make their intentional nontherapeutic use more difficult, less attractive, or less rewarding. No studies comparing the relative safety of these products are available. Whether using abuse-deterrent opioid products actually reduces overall opioid abuse remains to be determined. No opioid formulation prevents consumption of a large number of intact dosage units, the most common method of abuse.[33-35]

FULL AGONIST/REUPTAKE INHIBITORS

TAPENTADOL — Tapentadol is an oral opioid agonist and a norepinephrine reuptake inhibitor.[36] It is a schedule II controlled substance and is available in short-acting and extended-release formulations. The extended-release formulation appears to provide analgesic efficacy similar to that of extended-release oxycodone with fewer adverse GI effects.[37] Due to its serotonergic effects, it is contraindicated for use with or within 14 days of taking an MAO inhibitor.

TRAMADOL — An oral centrally-acting opioid agonist that weakly inhibits reuptake of norepinephrine and serotonin, tramadol is used to treat moderate to moderately severe pain. It is available alone and in combination with acetaminophen (*Ultracet,* and generics); the effectiveness of the combination for treatment of chronic pain is comparable to that of combinations of acetaminophen with codeine or oxycodone. The need for slow dose titration to decrease nausea and improve tolerability when initiating tramadol limits its use for treatment of acute pain. Tramadol may also be effective for treatment of neuropathic pain, but the supporting evidence is weak.[38]

Seizures have been reported with tramadol; patients with a history of seizures and those concomitantly taking a tricyclic antidepressant, a selective serotonin reuptake inhibitor, an MAO inhibitor, other opioids, or an antipsychotic drug may be at increased risk. Administration of naloxone for an overdose of tramadol may increase seizure risk. Tramadol is metabolized by CYP2D6 to a metabolite that is more active than tramadol itself; CYP2D6 poor metabolizers or those taking CYP2D6 inhibitors may not experience an analgesic effect. Concentrations of the active metabolite of tramadol may be higher in CYP2D6 ultra-rapid metabolizers, resulting in a higher incidence of adverse effects. Concurrent use of tramadol with drugs that inhibit CYP2D6 or 3A4 can increase tramadol levels and seizure risk.[20]

The FDA has issued warnings about cases of life-threatening respiratory depression and death that occurred in children who received tramadol. It is contraindicated for treatment of pain in children <12 years old and for treatment of pain after tonsillectomy or adenoidectomy in those <18 years old. Use of tramadol should be avoided in children 12-18 years old who are obese or have an increased risk of serious breathing problems and in breastfeeding women.[22] Tramadol is classified as a schedule IV controlled substance because it can cause psychological and physical dependence.

A PARTIAL AGONIST

The partial agonist **buprenorphine** is available in oral transmucosal *(Belbuca)* and parenteral formulations (*Buprenex*, and generics), and in a transdermal patch *(Butrans)* for treatment of pain. In some studies, oral or transdermal buprenorphine was effective in reducing pain in patients with chronic back pain.[39,40] Because of the low maximum dose of the patch (20 mcg/hr), it is not useful for treatment of severe cancer pain. Patients maintained on transdermal buprenorphine may require higher-than-normal doses of full opioid agonists during and for up to 48 hours following discontinuation of the patch.

Buprenorphine is also FDA-approved for maintenance treatment of opioid use disorder in oral transmucosal formulations (alone and in combination with the opioid antagonist naloxone), as a subdermal implant *(Probuphine),* and as a once-monthly injection *(Sublocade)*; it is safer than methadone because it has a ceiling on its respiratory depressant effect and a lower abuse potential, and is less likely to prolong the QT interval (in high doses, buprenorphine can prolong the QT interval).[5,41] Nausea, headache, dizziness, and somnolence are common adverse effects of buprenorphine.

MIXED AGONIST/ANTAGONISTS

The mixed agonist/antagonists **pentazocine** *(Talwin)*, **butorphanol**, and **nalbuphine** all have a ceiling on their analgesic effects and can precipitate withdrawal symptoms in patients physically dependent on full opioid agonists. All are less likely than full agonists to cause physical dependence, but none is entirely free of dependence liability.

1. Nonopioid drugs for pain. Med Lett Drugs Ther 2018; 60:24.
2. AK Chang et al. Effect of a single dose of oral opioid and nonopioid analgesics on acute extremity pain in the emergency department: a randomized clinical trial. JAMA 2017; 318:1661.
3. RA Deyo et al. Association between initial opioid prescribing patterns and subsequent long-term use among opioid-naïve patients: a statewide retrospective cohort study. J Gen Intern Med 2017; 32:21.
4. A Shah et al. Characteristics of initial prescription episodes and likelihood of long-term opioid use - United States, 2006-2015. MMWR Morb Mortal Wkly Rep 2017; 66:265.
5. Drugs for opioid use disorder. Med Lett Drugs Ther 2017; 59:89.
6. R Chou et al. The effectiveness and risks of long-term opioid therapy for chronic pain: a systematic review for a National Institutes of Health Pathways of Prevention Workshop. Ann Intern Med 2015; 162:276.
7. EE Krebs et al. Effect of opioid vs nonopioid medications on pain-related function in patients with chronic back pain or hip or knee osteoarthritis pain: the SPACE randomized clinical trial. JAMA 2018; 319:872.
8. D Dowell et al. CDC guideline for prescribing opioids for chronic pain – United States, 2016. MMWR Recomm Rep 2016; 65:1.
9. L Manchikanti et al. Responsible, safe, and effective prescription of opioids for chronic non-cancer pain: American Society of Interventional Pain Physicians (ASIPP) guidelines. Pain Physician 2017; 20(2S):S3.
10. AS Bohnert et al. A detailed exploration into the association of prescribed opioid dosage and overdose deaths among patients with chronic pain. Med Care 2016; 54:435.
11. New indications for modafinil (Provigil). Med Lett Drugs Ther 2004; 46:34.
12. Methylnaltrexone (Relistor) for opioid-induced constipation. Med Lett Drugs Ther 2008; 50:63.
13. Naloxegol (Movantik) for opioid-induced constipation. Med Lett Drugs Ther 2015; 57:135.
14. Naldemedine (Symproic) for opioid-induced constipation. Med Lett Drugs Ther 2017; 59:196.
15. Q Yang et al. Efficacy and adverse effects of transdermal fentanyl and sustained-release oral morphine in treating moderate-severe cancer pain in Chinese population: a systematic review and meta-analysis. J Exp Clin Cancer Res 2010; 29:67.
16. M Lee et al. A comprehensive review of opioid-induced hyperalgesia. Pain Physician 2011; 14:145.

17. MJ Brennan. The effect of opioid therapy on endocrine function. Am J Med 2013; 126:S12.
18. FDA Drug Safety Communication: FDA warns about several safety issues with opioid pain medicines; requires label changes. Available at: www.fda.gov/drugs/drugsafety/ucm489676.htm. Accessed March 29, 2018.
19. FDA Drug Safety Communication: FDA warns about serious risks and death when combining opioid pain or cough medicines with benzodiazepines; requires its strongest warning. August 31, 2016. Available at: www.fda.gov/drugs/drugsafety/ucm518473.htm. Accessed March 29, 2018.
20. Inhibitors and inducers of CYP enzymes and p-glycoprotein. Med Lett Drugs Ther 2017; September 18 (epub). Available at www.medicalletter.org/downloads/CYP_PGP_Tables.pdf. Accessed March 29, 2018.
21. VE Whiteman et al. Maternal opioid drug use during pregnancy and its impact on perinatal morbidity, mortality, and the costs of medical care in the United States. J Pregnancy 2014; 2014:906723.
22. FDA warns against use of codeine and tramadol in children and breastfeeding women. Med Lett Drugs Ther 2017; 59:86.
23. In brief: Heat and transdermal fentanyl. Med Lett Drugs Ther 2009; 51:64.
24. FDA Drug Safety Communication: FDA requiring color changes to Duragesic (fentanyl) pain patches to aid safety—emphasizing that accidental exposure to used patches can cause death. September 23, 2013. Available at: https://www.fda.gov/Drugs/DrugSafety/ucm368902.htm. Accessed March 29, 2018.
25. Extended-release hydrocodone (Zohydro ER) for pain. Med Lett Drugs Ther 2014; 56:45.
26. Extended-release hydrocodone (Hysingla ER) for pain. Med Lett Drugs Ther 2015; 57:71.
27. Extended-release hydromorphone (Exalgo) for pain. Med Lett Drugs Ther 2011; 53:62.
28. H Binsfeld et al. A randomized study to demonstrate noninferiority of once-daily OROS hydromorphone with twice-daily sustained-release oxycodone for moderate to severe chronic noncancer pain. Pain Pract 2010; 10:404.
29. E Bruera et al. Methadone versus morphine as a first-line strong opioid for cancer pain: a randomized, double-blind study. J Clin Oncol 2004; 22:185.
30. Centers for Disease Control and Prevention (CDC). Vital signs: risk for overdose from methadone used for pain relief—United States, 1999-2010. MMWR Morb Mortal Wkly Rep 2012; 61:493.
31. MJ Krantz et al. QTc interval screening in methadone treatment. Ann Intern Med 2009; 150:387.
32. Oral oxymorphone (Opana). Med Lett Drugs Ther 2007; 49:3.
33. Abuse-deterrent opioid formulations. Med Lett Drugs Ther 2015; 57:119.
34. Arymo ER – A new abuse-deterrent morphine formulation. Med Lett Drugs Ther 2017; 59:68.
35. A new abuse-deterrent opioid – Xtampza ER. Med Lett Drugs Ther 2016; 58:77.
36. Tapentadol (Nucynta) – a new analgesic. Med Lett Drugs Ther 2009; 51:61.
37. M Afilalo and B Morlion. Efficacy of tapentadol ER for managing moderate to severe chronic pain. Pain Physician 2013; 16:27.
38. RM Duehmke et al. Tramadol for neuropathic pain in adults. Cochrane Database Syst Rev 2017; 6:CD003726.

39. Transdermal buprenorphine (Butrans) for chronic pain. Med Lett Drugs Ther 2011; 53:31.
40. Buprenorphine buccal film (Belbuca) for chronic pain. Med Lett Drugs Ther 2016; 58:47.
41. Once-monthly subcutaneous buprenorphine (Sublocade) for opioid use disorder. Med Lett Drugs Ther 2018; 60:35.

Sunscreens

Original publication date — August 2018

Excessive exposure to ultraviolet (UV) radiation is associated with sunburn, photoaging, and skin cancer.[1,2] Sunscreens are widely used to reduce these risks, but some questions remain about their effectiveness and safety.

UVA and UVB — UV radiation capable of injuring the skin is classified based on wavelength as UVA1 (340-400 nm), UVA2 (320-340 nm), and UVB (290-320 nm). UVA, which makes up 95% of terrestrial UV radiation, penetrates the dermis and causes long-term damage. UVB, which is mostly absorbed in the epidermis, is largely responsible for the erythema of sunburn. Both UVA and UVB can cause photoaging and skin cancer. UVB is strongest at midday and is present primarily in late spring, summer, and early autumn in temperate climates. UVA is constant throughout the day and the year and, unlike UVB, is not filtered by clear glass.

SPF — Sun Protection Factor (SPF) is the ratio of the time required to develop a minimally detectable sunburn while wearing a sunscreen product to the time required without wearing the product. It represents the fraction of erythema-producing UV light (primarily UVB) that penetrates through the product to reach the skin. When properly applied, an SPF 15 sunscreen allows penetration of 1/15th (7%) of erythemogenic UV photons, an SPF 50 sunscreen transmits 1/50th (2%), and an SPF 100 sunscreen transmits 1/100th (1%). Accordingly, SPF 50 and 100 sunscreens are only moderately more protective than SPF 15 sunscreens: 98% or 99% vs 93%.

There is no specific rating system in the US for the amount of UVA protection provided by a sunscreen. The FDA allows sunscreens to be labeled "broad-spectrum" if they provide UVA and UVB protection and the UVA protection is proportional to the UVB protection. Broad-spectrum sunscreens with an SPF ≥15 can claim that they can reduce the risk of skin cancer and early skin aging if used as directed with other sun protection measures. The FDA and the US Preventive Services Task Force (USPSTF) both recommend use of a broad-spectrum sunscreen with an SPF ≥15.[3,4] The American Academy of Dermatology recommends use of a product with an SPF ≥30.[5]

SUNSCREEN ACTIVE INGREDIENTS — Organic – Several organic (chemical) sunscreens that absorb different wavelengths of UV light are approved by the FDA (see Table 1). Avobenzone is an effective UVA1 absorber and also absorbs some UVA2, but its efficacy decreases by about 60% after 60 minutes of exposure to sunlight due to photolability; the photostability of avobenzone is improved by combining it with other photostable UV filters. Octinoxate is a potent UVB absorber. Octisalate and homosalate are weak UVB absorbers; they are generally used with other agents for additional UVB protection. Octocrylene absorbs UVB and is photostable; when combined with other sunscreens, it can improve the photostability of the entire product. Ecamsule is photostable and absorbs both UVB and UVA2.[6]

Inorganic – The two FDA-approved inorganic (physical) sunscreens, zinc oxide and titanium dioxide, prevent UVB, UVA1, and UVA2 penetration. Micronized (nanoparticle) formulations that improve cosmetic acceptability are now widely used; they are less visible on the skin, but may also be less effective.[7]

EFFECTIVENESS — In the amounts customarily applied to skin, no sunscreen product provides the labeled degree of protection. The FDA

Table 1. FDA-Approved Sunscreens	
Sunscreen	**UV Protection**
Organic	
PABA Derivatives	
PABA (para-aminobenzoic acid)	UVB
Padimate O (octyl dimethyl PABA)	UVB
Cinnamates	
Cinoxate	UVB
Octinoxate (octyl methoxycinnamate)	UVB
Salicylates	
Homosalate	UVB
Octisalate (octyl salicylate)	UVB
Trolamine salicylate	UVB
Benzophenones	
Dioxybenzone (benzophenone-8)	UVB, UVA2
Oxybenzone (benzophenone-3)	UVB, UVA2
Sulisobenzone (benzophenone-4)	UVB, UVA2
Others	
Avobenzone (butyl methoxydibenzoyl methane, *Parsol 1789*)	UVA1[1]
Ecamsule[2] (terephthalylidene dicamphor sulfonic acid)	UVB, UVA2
Ensulizone (phenylbenzimidazole sulfonic acid)	UVB
Meradimate (menthyl anthranilate)	UVA2
Octocrylene	UVB
Inorganic	
Titanium dioxide	UVB, UVA2, UVA1
Zinc oxide	UVB, UVA2, UVA1
UVB = 290-320 nm; UVA2 = 320-340 nm; UVA1 = 340-400 nm; 1. May also provide UVA2 protection. 2. *Meroxyl SX*, patented by L'Oreal.	

requires that the SPF be determined after applying 2 mg/cm^2 of the product, a very thick layer. At 2 mg/cm^2, a 4-ounce container provides only 2-4 whole body applications for an adult. Studies have shown that consumers usually apply 0.5-1.0 mg/cm^2 or less. Applied in these amounts, sunscreens (SPF 30-100) provide an actual SPF that is about 25% of the labeled SPF.[8] Nevertheless, studies have found that long-term daily sunscreen use combined with other sun-protective measures

Table 2. Some Sunscreen Products[1]	
Product[2]	**Formulation**
SPF 15	
Anthelios SX SPF 15 (La Roche-Posay)	Cream (3.4 oz)
Badger Active SPF 15 (W.S. Badger)	Cream (2.9 fl oz)
Banana Boat Protective Dry Oil SPF 15 (Edgewell)	Spray (6.0 fl oz)
Coppertone Sport SPF 15 (Bayer)	Spray (6.0 fl oz)
Hawaiian Tropic Sheer Touch SPF 15 (Edgewell)	Lotion (8.0 fl oz)
No-Ad SPF 15 (No-Ad)	Lotion (16 fl oz)
Panama Jack SPF 15 (Panama Jack)	Spray (6.0 fl oz)
Sun Bum 15 (Sun Bum)	Lotion (8.0 fl oz)
SPF 30(+)	
Australian Gold Botanical SPF 30 (Australian Gold)	Lotion (5.0 fl oz)
Aveeno Active Naturals Protect + Hydrate SPF 30 (Johnson & Johnson)	Lotion (3.0 fl oz)
Badger Sport SPF 35 (W.S. Badger)	Cream (2.9 fl oz)
Banana Boat Sport Performance SPF 30 (Edgewell)	Spray (6.0 fl oz)
Blue Lizard Australian Regular SPF 30+ (Crown)	Lotion (8.75 fl oz)
Coppertone Sport SPF 30 (Bayer)	Spray (6.0 fl oz)
Kiss My Face Sun Spray Lotion SPF 30 (Kiss My Face)	Lotion (8.0 fl oz)
Neutrogena Cool Dry Sport SPF 30 (Neutrogena)	Spray (5.0 fl oz)
SPF 50(+)	
Anthelios SPF 60 Melt-In Milk (La Roche-Posay)	Lotion (5.0 fl oz)
Babyganics SPF 50+ (Babyganics)	Spray (6.0 fl oz)
Banana Boat Kids Sport SPF 50+ (Edgewell)	Lotion (6 fl oz)
Banana Boat Sun Comfort SPF 50+ (Edgewell)	Spray (5.0 fl oz)

1. Sunscreens are also found in many cosmetic products including facial moisturizers, lip balms, foundations, and powders and sprays marketed for application over makeup.
2. Individual stores may carry their own brand of sunscreen.

Active Ingredients	UV Protection	Cost[3]
Avobenzone 2%, ecamsule[4] 2%, octocrylene 10%	UVB/UVA2/UVA1	$34.00
Zinc oxide 10%	UVB/UVA2/UVA1	13.60
Avobenzone 1.5%, homosalate 5%, octocrylene 3.5%	UVB/UVA1[5]	10.99
Avobenzone 2%, octisalate 4.5%, octocrylene 7%	UVB/UVA1[5]	11.49
Avobenzone 1.5%, homosalate 3%, octisalate 4.5%, octocrylene 3%	UVB/UVA1[5]	11.79
Avobenzone 1.2%, homosalate 7.5%, octisalate 5%	UVB/UVA1[5]	7.57
Octinoxate 5%, octisalate 3%, oxybenzone 2%	UVB/UVA2	10.99
Avobenzone 2%, homosalate 5%, octisalate 2%, octocrylene 1.85%, oxybenzone 3%	UVB/UVA2/UVA1	16.00
Titanium dioxide 3%, zinc oxide 3%	UVB/UVA2/UVA1	12.99
Avobenzone 3%, homosalate 8%, octisalate 4%, octocrylene 4%, oxybenzone 5%	UVB/UVA2/UVA1	11.99
Zinc oxide 22.5%	UVB/UVA2/UVA1	13.60
Avobenzone 1%, octocrylene 7.7%, oxybenzone 3%	UVB/UVA2/UVA1	9.99
Octinoxate 7.5%, octocrylene 2%, oxybenzone 3%, zinc oxide 6%	UVB/UVA2/UVA1	22.99
Avobenzone 3%, octisalate 4.5%, octocrylene 7%, oxybenzone 4%	UVB/UVA2/UVA1	10.49
Octinoxate 7.5%, octisalate 5%, zinc oxide 1.7%	UVB/UVA2/UVA1	13.69
Avobenzone 3%, homosalate 8%, octisalate 5%, octocrylene 4%, oxybenzone 5%	UVB/UVA2/UVA1	11.49
Avobenzone 3%, homosalate 10.72%, octisalate 3.21%, octocrylene 6%, oxybenzone 3.86%	UVB/UVA2/UVA1	36.00
Zinc oxide 11.2%, octinoxate 7.5%, octisalate 5%	UVB/UVA2/UVA1	11.99
Titanium dioxide 4.5%, zinc oxide 6.5%	UVB/UVA2/UVA1	11.49
Avobenzone 3%, homosalate 10%, octisalate 5%, octocrylene 3%, oxybenzone 4%	UVB/UVA2/UVA1	11.49

3. Prices according to walgreens.com. Accessed July 12, 2018.
4. *Meroxyl SX*, patented by L'Oreal.
5. May also provide UVA2 protection.

Continued on next page

Table 2. Some Sunscreen Products[1] (continued)	
Product[2]	**Formulation**
SPF 50(+) (continued)	
Bull Frog Land Sport Quik Gel SPF 50 (Chattem)	Gel (1.5 oz)
Coppertone Kids Tear Free SPF 50 (Bayer)	Lotion (6.0 fl oz)
Neutrogena Beach Defense Water + Sun Protection Stick SPF 50+ (Neutrogena)	Stick (1.5 oz)
No-Ad Sport Stick SPF 50 (No-Ad)	Stick (1.5 oz)

can reduce the risk of non-melanoma skin cancer and can reduce other adverse effects of UV exposure such as photoaging.[9-11]

Prevention of Melanoma – Fair skin, use of tanning beds, and a history of sunburn are associated with increased melanoma risk.[4] In a recently published population-based, case-control study in 603 Australian adults 18-39 years old with a first primary cutaneous melanoma diagnosis and 1088 controls 18-44 years old, regular sunscreen use was associated with a reduced risk of cutaneous melanoma.[12] In a prospective trial, 1621 Australians 25-75 years old were randomized to use an SPF 16 sunscreen either daily or in a discretionary manner (generally 0-2 times weekly) for 4 years. Compared with discretionary users, daily sunscreen users had half as many new primary melanomas (11 vs 22) and a 73% reduction in invasive melanomas (3 vs 11) 14 years after randomization.[13]

SAFETY — All organic sunscreens, especially oxybenzone, can cause contact allergic and photoallergic reactions, but these reactions are uncommon.[14] Estrogen-like activity has been reported *in vitro* and in some animal studies. These agents can penetrate the epidermis and small amounts can be absorbed systemically; detectable levels have been reported in human plasma, urine, breast milk, amniotic fluid, and fetal and cord blood.[15-17] Whether such exposure could result in hormonal alterations or other adverse effects in humans is unclear.[18,19]

Active Ingredients	UV Protection	Cost[3]
Avobenzone 3%, homosalate 15%, octisalate 5%, octocrylene 10%, oxybenzone 6%	UVB/UVA2/UVA1	$12.49
Octinoxate 7.5%, octisalate 5%, zinc oxide 14.5%	UVB/UVA2/UVA1	12.49
Avobenzone 3%, homosalate 15%, octisalate 5%, octocrylene 10%, oxybenzone 3%	UVB/UVA2/UVA1	11.49
Avobenzone 3%, homosalate 10%, octisalate 5%, octocrylene 10%, oxybenzone 3%	UVB/UVA2/UVA1	6.99

An Australian government review of the safety of titanium dioxide and zinc oxide nanoparticles concluded that these microfine particles do not penetrate or minimally penetrate the stratum corneum and underlying layers of skin, suggesting that systemic absorption and toxicity are unlikely.[20]

Environmental Safety – In Hawaii, legislation was recently passed banning the sale of sunscreens that contain oxybenzone and/or octinoxate because they can cause coral bleaching.[21] Detectable concentrations of sunscreens have been observed in some fish species and adverse reproductive effects have been reported.[22]

USE IN INFANTS AND CHILDREN — Sunscreen use is generally recommended for children >6 months old during any sun exposure that might burn unprotected skin. Inorganic sunscreens are less likely than organic sunscreens to cause irritation and sensitization.[23]

VITAMIN D AND SUNSCREENS — Most people require only 2-8 minutes of unprotected exposure to summer sun to maximize synthesis of vitamin D_3. Whether sunscreen use could lead to vitamin D_3 deficiency is unclear.

APPLICATION — For maximum efficacy, sunscreen should be applied about 15-30 minutes before sun exposure and reapplied at least every two hours and after swimming or sweating. Water-resistant sunscreens remain effective for 40 or 80 minutes while swimming or sweating; no sunscreens are waterproof. For maximum effect, approximately one teaspoon of sunscreen should be applied to the face and neck and one to each arm; two teaspoons should be applied to the torso and two to each leg.[24]

When using both a sunscreen and an insect repellent, the sunscreen should be applied first. Applying the insect repellent *N,N-diethyl-m-* tolumide (DEET) after sunscreen has been shown to reduce the SPF of the sunscreen, but applying sunscreen second may increase absorption of DEET. The CDC does not recommend use of products that combine a sunscreen with an insect repellent because the sunscreen may need to be reapplied more often and in greater amounts than the repellent.[25]

PROTECTIVE CLOTHING — Clothing can block UV exposure. Factors that affect the level of UV protection from clothing include fabric color, fabric type, and tightness of the weave. The ultraviolet protection factor (UPF) is a measure of how effective a fabric is at blocking UV radiation; a rating of 15-24 indicates good protection, 25-39 very good protection, and 40-50 excellent protection. Washing clothes with *RIT Sun Guard* can confer a UPF of 30.

CONCLUSION — Routine application of adequate amounts of a broad-spectrum sunscreen with an SPF ≥ 15 protects against sunburn, photoaging, non-melanoma skin cancer, and probably melanoma as well. Whether systemic absorption of small amounts of sunscreen ingredients could be harmful remains to be determined, but currently available data suggest that the benefits far outweigh the risks.

1. U Panich et al. Ultraviolet radiation-induced skin aging: the role of DNA damage and oxidative stress in epidermal stem cell damage mediated skin aging. Stem Cells Int 2016; 2016:7370642.
2. M Arnold et al. Global burden of cutaneous melanoma attributable to ultraviolet radiation in 2012. Int J Cancer 2018 April 16 (epub).
3. Questions and answers: FDA announces new requirements for over-the-counter (OTC) sunscreen products marketed in the U.S. June 23, 2011. Available at: www.fda.gov/

drugs/resourcesforyou/consumers/buyingusingmedicinesafely/understandingover-the-countermedicines/ucm258468.htm. Accessed August 2, 2018.

4. US Preventive Services Task Force. Behavorial counseling to prevent skin cancer: US Preventive Services Task Force recommendation statement. JAMA 2018; 319:1134.

5. AAD statement on the safety of sunscreen. American Academy of Dermatology. October 22, 2015. Available at: www.aad.org/media/news-releases/aad-statement-on-the-safety-of-sunscreen. Accessed August 2, 2018.

6. A new sunscreen agent. Med Lett Drugs Ther 2007; 49:41.

7. JB Mancuso et al. Sunscreens: an update. Am J Clin Dermatol 2017; 18:643.

8. H Ou-Yang et al. High-SPF sunscreens (SPF ≥70) may provide ultraviolet protection above minimal recommended levels by adequately compensating for lower sunscreen user application amounts. J Am Acad Dermatol 2012; 67:1220.

9. JC van der Pols et al. Prolonged prevention of squamous cell carcinoma of the skin by regular sunscreen use. Cancer Epidemiol Biomarkers Prev 2006; 15:2546.

10. C Ulrich et al. Prevention of non-melanoma skin cancer in organ transplant patients by regular use of a sunscreen: a 24 month, prospective, case-control study. Br J Dermatol 2009; 161 (suppl 3:78).

11. MC Hughes et al. Sunscreen and prevention of skin aging: a randomized trial. Ann Intern Med 2013; 158:781.

12. CG Watts et al. Sunscreen use and melanoma risk among young Australian adults. JAMA Dermatol 2018 July 18 (epub).

13. AC Green et al. Reduced melanoma after regular sunscreen use: randomized trial follow-up. J Clin Oncol 2011; 29:257.

14. AR Heurung et al. Adverse reactions to sunscreen agents: epidemiology, responsible irritants and allergans, clinical characteristics, and management. Dermatitis 2014; 25:289.

15. NR Janjua et al. Systemic absorption of the sunscreens benzophenone-3, octyl-methoxycinnamate, and 3-(4-methyl-benzylidene) camphor after whole-body topical application and reproductive hormone levels in humans. J Invest Dermatol 2004; 123:57.

16. GM Buck Louis et al. Urinary concentrations of benzophenone-type ultraviolet radiation filters and couples' fecundity. Am J Epidemiol 2014; 180:1168.

17. H Krause et al. Presence of benzophenones commonly used as UV filters and absorbers in paired maternal and fetal samples. Environ Int 2018; 110:51.

18. SQ Wang et al. Safety of oxybenzone: putting numbers into perspective. Arch Dermatol 2011; 147:865.

19. JA Ruszkiewicz et al. Neurotoxic effect of active ingredients in sunscreen products, a contemporary review. Toxicol Rep 2017; 4:245.

20. Australian Government Department of Health. Therapeutic Goods Administration. Literature review on the safety of titanium dioxide and zinc oxide nanoparticles in sunscreens. January 11, 2017. Available at: www.tga.gov.au/node/4309. Accessed August 2, 2018.

21. CA Downs et al. Toxicopathological effects of the sunscreen UV filter, oxybenzone (benzophenone-3) on coral planulae and cultured primary cells and its environmental contamination in Hawaii and the U.S. Virgin Islands. Arch Environ Contam Toxicol 2016; 70:265.

22. SL Schneider and HW Lim. Review of environmental effects of oxybenzone and other sunscreen active ingredients. J Am Acad Dermatol 2018 June 28 (epub).

Vaccines for Travelers

Original publication date – November 2018

Persons planning to travel outside the US should be up to date on routine vaccines and, depending on their destination, duration of travel, and planned activities, may also receive certain travel-specific vaccines. Tickborne encephalitis and dengue vaccines, which are not available in the US, are reviewed in a separate article available online. Detailed advice for travel to specific destinations is available from the Centers for Disease Control and Prevention (CDC) at www.cdc.gov/travel/destinations/list. Recommendations for administration of vaccines as part of routine adult immunization are discussed in a separate issue.[1]

TIMING OF VACCINE ADMINISTRATION

Multiple inactivated and/or live-attenuated vaccines can generally be given on the same day at different sites without decreasing antibody responses or increasing the risk of adverse effects. If two live-attenuated vaccines are not administered on the same day, the second one should generally be given at least one month after the first. An interrupted vaccine series does not have to be restarted; there is no maximum interval between doses of a primary series.[2]

Immunocompromised or pregnant patients generally should not receive live vaccines, although the benefit might outweigh the risk in some situations.[3]

VACCINES

CHOLERA — Cholera is endemic in many countries in Africa and South and Southeast Asia. In recent years, most outbreaks have been caused by toxigenic strains of *Vibrio cholerae* serogroup O1. Cases caused by serogroup O139 have occurred in a few areas in Asia.

For most tourists, the risk of cholera is very low. Travelers who might have a higher risk of exposure include those who plan to work in refugee camps, in outbreak settings, or as healthcare providers, and those visiting friends and relatives or staying for extended periods in affected areas.

Recommendations – The US Advisory Committee on Immunization Practices (ACIP) recommends vaccination for persons 18-64 years old traveling to areas with endemic or epidemic cholera caused by toxigenic *V. cholerae* serogroup O1, including areas with cholera activity within the last year that are prone to recurrences of cholera epidemics.[4]

The Vaccine – *Vaxchora*, a single-dose, oral, live-attenuated cholera vaccine, is FDA-licensed to protect against disease caused by toxigenic *V. cholerae* serogroup O1 (but not serogroup O139 or other non-O1 serogroups) in adults 18-64 years old. It should be taken at least 10 days before potential cholera exposure.[5]

In a randomized trial, volunteers were challenged with wild-type *V. cholerae* serogroup O1 10 days or 3 months after vaccination; the seroconversion rate was 89% at 10 days and 90% at 180 days after vaccination.Vaccine efficacy against moderate or severe diarrhea was 90% at 10 days and 80% at 3 months.[6]

HEPATITIS A — Hepatitis A virus (HAV) is common in countries where sanitation is poor and access to clean water is limited, including many parts of Africa, Asia, Central and South America, and Eastern Europe. Areas with low levels of endemic HAV transmission include Western Europe, Japan, New Zealand, and Australia. HAV vaccination has been part of routine childhood immunization in the US since 2006.

Recommendations – HAV vaccine is recommended by the ACIP for all unvaccinated travelers going to countries with intermediate or high HAV endemicity.[7] However, there is a potential risk of foodborne HAV infection even in countries with low endemicity; some experts advise all persons traveling outside the US to consider hepatitis A vaccination regardless of their destination.

The Vaccines – Monovalent HAV vaccines *(Havrix, Vaqta)* are usually administered in 2 IM doses at least 6 months apart. Antibodies reach protective levels 2-4 weeks after the first dose. Even when exposure to the virus occurs sooner than 4 weeks after vaccination, the traveler is usually protected because the hepatitis A incubation period is relatively long (average 28 days). Immunocompromised patients, who have reduced seroconversion rates after the first dose of HAV vaccine, may benefit from an extra priming dose; in a study in adults with drug-induced immunosuppression given 2 doses 4 weeks apart, the seroprotection rate at 2 months was 84%.[8] A series started with one of the two monovalent hepatitis A vaccines may be completed with the other, or (in adults) with the combination hepatitis A/hepatitis B virus vaccine *(Twinrix)*. A second dose given up to 11 years after the first has produced protective antibody levels.[9]

For older adults, immunocompromised patients, and those with chronic liver disease or other chronic medical conditions who will be traveling to an endemic area in ≤2 weeks, one dose of immune globulin *(GamaSTAN S/D)* should be given in addition to the initial dose of vaccine. Infants <6 months old and persons who elect not to receive the vaccine should receive a single dose of immune globulin before travel. Infants 6-11 months old may receive a single dose of vaccine before travel instead of immune globulin, followed by a complete 2-dose series beginning at ≥12 months of age; the rationale for off-label use of the vaccine in this age group is that HAV and live-attenuated measles, mumps, and rubella (MMR)

Table 1. Some Vaccines for Travelers

Vaccines	Adult Dose	Pediatric Dose
Cholera		
Vaxchora (PaxVax)	18-64 yrs: 100 mL PO (reconstituted)	Not approved for <18 yrs
Hepatitis A		
Havrix (GSK)	1 mL IM (1440 EL.U.)	1-18 yrs: 0.5 mL IM (720 EL.U)
Vaqta (Merck)	1 mL IM (50 units)	1-18 yrs: 0.5 mL IM (25 units)
Hepatitis B		
Engerix-B (GSK)	1 mL IM (20 mcg) 1 mL IM (10 mcg)	Birth-19 yrs: 0.5 mL IM (10 mcg)
Recombivax-HB (Merck)		Birth-19 yrs: 0.5 mL IM (5 mcg)
Heplisav-B (Dynavax)	0.5 mL IM (20 mcg)	Not approved for <18 yrs
Hepatitis A/B		
Twinrix (GSK)[5]	1 mL IM (720 EL.U./20 mcg)	Not approved for <18 yrs
Japanese encephalitis		
Ixiaro (Valneva)	0.5 mL IM	2 mos-<3 yrs: 0.25 mL IM ≥3 yrs: 0.5 mL IM

EL.U. = ELISA Units
1. Protection probably lasts at least 12 months after a single dose.
2. An alternate schedule is 3 doses given at 0, 1, and 2 months, followed by a fourth dose at 12 months.
3. An accelerated schedule (0, 7, and 21-30 days, followed by a booster dose at 12 months) that is FDA-approved for use with *Twinrix* may also be used, if necessary, with hepatitis B vaccine.
4. An alternate schedule for adolescents 11-15 years old is 0 and 4-6 months.
5. Contains the same antigenic components as pediatric *Havrix* (hepatitis A) and *Engerix-B* (hepatitis B). It can be used to complete an immunization series started with monovalent hepatitis A and B vaccines.

Primary Schedule	Duration of Protection
Single dose	▸ Probably at least 6 mos
0 and 6-12 mos 0 and 6-18 mos	▸ Probably lifelong after completion of primary series[1]
0, 1, and 6 mos[2,3] 0, 1, and 6 mos[3,4] 0 and 1 mo	▸ Probably lifelong after completion of primary series
0, 1, and 6 mos (alternative: 0, 7, and 21-30 days)	▸ Booster recommended at 12 mos with accelerated schedule; otherwise probably lifelong after completion of primary series
0 and 28 days[6] (alternative: 0 and 7 days for adults 18-65 yrs old)	▸ A single booster ≥11 mos after completion of primary series is recommended for those ≥14 mos old with ongoing risk[7,8]

6. For last-minute travelers, one double dose of the vaccine (not FDA-approved) has been shown to provide 60% protection for at least one month (E Schuller et al. Vaccine 2009; 27:2188).
7. One study found that a single dose of *Ixiaro* effectively boosted immunity in travelers previously vaccinated with *JE-Vax* (EO Erra et al. Vaccine 2013; 32:119), but the ACIP recommends that adults previously vaccinated with *JE-Vax* receive a primary series of *Ixiaro* (MMWR Morb Mortal Wkly Rep 2011; 60:661).
8. In an observational study in adults who had completed a primary series of *Ixiaro*, the seroprotection rate was 96% six years after a booster dose (M Paulke-Korinck et al. Vaccine 2015; 33:3600).

Continued on next page

Table 1. Some Vaccines for Travelers (continued)		
Vaccines	**Adult Dose**	**Pediatric Dose**
Meningococcal		
Menveo (GSK)	0.5 mL IM (10 mcg serogroup A, 5 mcg serogroup C, Y, W135)	≥2 mos: 0.5 mL IM (10 mcg serogroup A, 5 mcg serogroup C, Y, W135)
Menactra (Sanofi Pasteur)	0.5 mL IM (4 mcg of each antigen)	≥9 mos: 0.5 mL IM (4 mcg of each antigen)
Polio		
Ipol (Sanofi Pasteur)	0.5 mL IM or SC	≥6 wks: 0.5 mL IM or SC
Rabies		
Imovax (Sanofi Pasteur)	1 mL IM (≥2.5 IU of rabies antigen)	≥Birth: 1 mL IM (≥2.5 IU of rabies antigen)
RabAvert (GSK)	1 mL IM (≥2.5 IU of rabies antigen)	≥Birth: 1 mL IM (≥2.5 IU of rabies antigen)
Typhoid		
Vivotif (PaxVax)	1 cap PO (contains 2.0-10.0x10^9 viable CFU of *S. typhi* Ty21a)	≥6 yrs: 1 cap PO (contains 2.0-10.0x10^9 viable CFU of *S. typhi* Ty21a)
Typhim Vi (Sanofi Pasteur)	0.5 mL IM (25 mcg of Vi polysaccharide)	≥2 yrs: 0.5 mL IM (25 mcg of Vi polysaccharide)
Yellow Fever		
YF-Vax (Sanofi Pasteur)[19]	0.5 mL SC (4.74 log$_{10}$ plaque forming units of 17D204 attenuated YF virus)	≥9 mos: 0.5 mL SC (4.74 log$_{10}$ plaque forming units of 17D204 attenuated YF virus)

CFU = colony-forming units
9. The second dose should be given at age 12 months and ≥3 months after the first, but can be administered as early as 8 weeks after the first dose if needed before travel.
10. For children 2-5 years old at continued high risk, a second dose may be administered 2 months after the first.
11. Although FDA-licensed only for persons <56 years old, the CDC states that *Menveo* or *Menactra* may be administered to travelers aged ≥56 years.
12. Repeat after 3 years for children vaccinated at <7 years of age.
13. The second dose can be administered 8 weeks after the first if required before travel.
14. If primary series completed. Previously unvaccinated adults should receive 2 doses 4-8 weeks apart, followed by a third dose 6-12 months after the second.
15. Alternative for previously unvaccinated children ≥6 weeks old is a primary series consisting of 3 doses given ≥4 weeks apart, followed by a fourth dose 6 months after the third.

Primary Schedule	Duration of Protection
2 mos: 2, 4, 6, and 12 mos 7-23 mos: 0 and 3 mos[9] ≥2 yrs: single dose[10,11]	► Repeat every 5 yrs[12] if ongoing risk
9-23 mos: 0 and 3 mos[13] ≥2 yrs: single dose[11]	
Adults: single dose[14] Children: 2, 4, 6-18 mos and 4-6 yrs[15]	► Boosters may be required for long-term travel to polio-affected countries
0, 7, and 21 or 28 days[16] 0, 7, and 21 or 28 days[16]	► Routine boosters generally not necessary; for those engaging in frequent high-risk activities (cavers, veterinarians, laboratory workers), serologic testing is recommended every 6 mos with booster doses if low levels[17]
1 cap every other day x 4 doses[18]	► Repeat every 5 yrs if ongoing risk
Single dose	► Repeat every 2 yrs (3 yrs in Canada) if ongoing risk
Single dose	► Possibly lifelong

16. Regimen for pre-exposure prophylaxis (PrEP). The World Health Organization (WHO) recommends a 2-dose PrEP schedule on days 0 and 7, and states that, in case of time constraints, a single dose will likely confer some protection, but those who have received 1 dose should receive a 2nd dose as soon as possible and within 1 year (WHO. Rabies vaccines: WHO position pager – April 2018. Weekly Epidemiological Record 2018; 93:201. Available at www.who.int/wer/2018/en. Accessed November 8, 2018). If a previously vaccinated traveler is exposed to a potentially rabid animal, post-exposure prophylaxis (PEP) with 2 additional vaccine doses 3 days apart should be given as soon as possible.
17. Minimal acceptable antibody level is complete virus neutralization at a 1:5 serum dilution by the rapid fluorescent focus inhibition test.
18. Taken about 1 hour before a meal with a cold or luke-warm drink.
19. *YF-Vax* is currently (November 2018) out of stock. Supplies are expected to be available by the middle of 2019. Another single-dose, live vaccine (*Stamaril*), which is licensed in Europe, is available at some US clinics (www.cdc.gov/travel/page/search-for-stamaril-clinics).

vaccines can be administered simultaneously, but MMR vaccine cannot be administered with immune globulin.[10] The recommended dosage of immune globulin, which was increased in 2017, varies according to the duration of travel: 0.1 mL/kg for up to one month of travel; 0.2 mL/kg for up to 2 months; 0.2 mL/kg every 2 months for longer travel.[11]

HEPATITIS B — Hepatitis B surface antigen (HbsAg) prevalence is generally high in sub-Saharan Africa and the Western Pacific region and low in most countries in the Americas, Western Europe, Japan, and Australia.[12] Hepatitis B virus (HBV) vaccine is part of routine childhood immunization in the US.

Recommendations – HBV vaccine is recommended by the ACIP for all travelers going to areas with intermediate or high prevalence of chronic HBV infection.[9] The risk for most travelers is low. Travelers who engage in behaviors that increase the risk of transmission, such as injection drug use, unprotected sexual contact with new partners, dental treatment, skin perforation practices (tattoos, acupuncture, ear piercing), or medical tourism involving invasive medical treatment, should receive the HBV vaccine regardless of their destination.[13]

The Vaccines – Three monovalent HBV vaccines are available in the US *(Engerix-B, Heplisav-B, Recombivax)*. *Heplisav-B* is a 2-dose vaccine that is only FDA-licensed for use in adults. The other vaccines are usually administered in 3 doses. In randomized clinical trials, seroprotection rates with 2 doses of *Heplisav-B* were significantly higher than those with 3 doses of *Engerix-B*.[14]

The ACIP recommends using the same vaccine for all doses of a hepatitis B series, but an interrupted series does not have to be restarted if the same vaccine is not available. Two doses of *Heplisav-B* can be used to complete a series started with a single dose of another monovalent vaccine or the combination HAV/HBV vaccine. One dose of *Heplisav-B* can be used as part of a 3-dose series.[15]

INFLUENZA— Influenza may be a risk in temperate areas of the Southern Hemisphere from April to September and of the Northern Hemisphere from October to March, and in the tropics year-round. Increased risk has been associated with travel in large tour groups and on cruise ships and airplanes, participation in mass gatherings, and staying abroad for >30 days. Persons traveling to East and Southeast Asia appear to have a higher risk of acquiring influenza than those traveling to other regions.[16]

Recommendations – The ACIP recommends routine annual vaccination against seasonal influenza for everyone ≥6 months old; detailed recommendations are included in a separate issue.[17]

Travelers not vaccinated during the preceding Northern Hemisphere influenza season should consider being vaccinated before going to the Southern Hemisphere during that region's influenza season or to the tropics in any season, or when traveling in a group with persons from the Southern Hemisphere during their influenza season.[18]

The Vaccines – Northern Hemisphere influenza vaccine is usually available in the US from August until the end of June. The vaccine formulations may be the same in the Northern and Southern Hemispheres. If they are different, high-risk patients from the Northern Hemisphere who travel to the Southern Hemisphere during that region's influenza season could consider vaccination prior to departure with a US-licensed Southern Hemisphere formulation *(Fluzone Quadrivalent Southern Hemisphere)*, if available, or vaccination upon arrival in the Southern Hemisphere. Serum antibody levels peak about 2 weeks after vaccination in most adults.

JAPANESE ENCEPHALITIS — Japanese encephalitis is an uncommon but potentially fatal mosquito-borne viral disease that occurs in rural Asia, especially near pig farms and rice paddies. It is usually seasonal (May-October), but may occur year-round in tropical regions. The incidence in travelers has been very low.[19]

Recommendations – Vaccination is recommended for travelers who expect a long stay (≥1 month) in endemic areas or heavy exposure to mosquitoes (such as adventure travelers) during the transmission season. Vaccination should be considered for travelers spending <1 month in endemic areas during the transmission season if they will be sleeping without air conditioning, screens, or bed nets, or spending considerable time outside in rural or agricultural areas, especially in the evening or at night.[20]

The Vaccine – *Ixiaro*, an inactivated Vero cell culture-derived vaccine, is the only Japanese encephalitis vaccine currently available in the US.[21] It is licensed by the FDA for use in adults and children ≥2 months old.[22] *Ixiaro* is usually given in 2 doses 28 days apart. The FDA has now approved an accelerated schedule (0 and 7 days) of *Ixiaro* that can be used as an alternative for last-minute adult travelers ≤65 years old. In a randomized trial in healthy adults 18-65 years old, the accelerated schedule was noninferior to the standard schedule in terms of immunogenicity and safety at one month and one year after vaccination.[23,24]

In an observational study, 96% of adults who had completed a 2-dose primary series of *Ixiaro* and received one booster dose 15 months later were still seroprotected 6 years after their booster dose.[25]

A single dose of *Ixiaro* has been shown to effectively boost antibody levels in persons vaccinated with a previously available vaccine *(JE-Vax)*, but the duration of protection is unknown; the ACIP recommends that persons previously vaccinated with *JE-Vax* who require continued protection receive a 2-dose primary series of *Ixiaro*.

MEASLES — Travel has been associated with importation of measles virus from other countries where it is endemic or large outbreaks are occurring, leading to outbreaks in the US, primarily among unvaccinated persons.[26]

Recommendations – The CDC recommends vaccination against measles for all persons without evidence of immunity, particularly international travelers. Children 6-11 months old should receive one MMR dose before traveling; they will still need 2 more doses of a measles-containing vaccine for routine immunization, beginning at ≥12 months of age. Previously unvaccinated children ≥12 months old, adolescents, and adults (born in 1957 or later [1970 in Canada]) should receive 2 doses of a measles-containing vaccine at least 28 days apart.[27,28]

The Vaccine – The measles vaccine is available as a live-attenuated vaccine in combination with mumps and rubella (MMR; *M-M-R-II*) or with mumps, rubella, and varicella (MMRV; *ProQuad;* approved only for children 12 months-12 years old).

MENINGOCOCCAL — Outbreaks of meningococcal disease can occur anywhere in the world, but they are most common in the African "meningitis belt" (semi-arid areas of sub-Saharan Africa extending from Senegal and Guinea eastward to Ethiopia). Recent outbreaks have primarily been due to *Neisseria meningitidis* serogroups C and W.

The Vaccines – Two quadrivalent inactivated vaccines against *N. meningitidis* serogroups A, C, W, and Y (MenACWY; *Menactra; Menveo*) are available in the US.[29,30] Both contain meningococcal capsular polysaccharides conjugated to a protein carrier. A third unconjugated quadrivalent polysaccharide vaccine *(Menomune)* is no longer available in the US.

Persons traveling to Saudi Arabia during the Hajj or Umrah must present proof of immunization with MenACWY. The vaccine must be administered no fewer than 10 days and no more than 3 years before travel if the previously available polysaccharide vaccine was used and no more than 5 years before if the conjugate vaccine was used.[31]

Two vaccines against *N. meningitidis* serogroup B (MenB; *Trumenba; Bexsero*) are available for use in persons 10-25 years old. MenB vaccine is not routinely recommended for travel unless an outbreak has been reported.

Recommendations – Vaccination with MenACWY is recommended for travelers going anywhere in the meningitis belt during the dry season (December to June), and should also be considered for areas where outbreaks of *N. meningitidis* are occurring, particularly for travelers who will have prolonged contact with the local population, such as those living in a dormitory, military institution, or refugee camp, or working in a healthcare setting.[28]

PNEUMOCOCCAL — The incidence of pneumococcal disease is higher in some developing countries than in the US. Pneumococcal vaccination has been part of routine childhood immunization in the US since 2010.

The Vaccines – Two pneumococcal vaccines are available in the US: PCV13 *(Prevnar 13)*, a conjugate vaccine that contains 13 serotypes of pneumococcus, and PPSV23 *(Pneumovax 23)*, a 23-valent pneumococcal polysaccharide vaccine.

Recommendations – Travelers should be up to date on pneumococcal vaccination. It is recommended for healthy adults ≥65 years old and for some persons <65 years old with certain immunocompromising conditions or other risk factors (e.g., smoking and chronic diseases such as diabetes). Healthy adults ≥65 years old who have not previously received either vaccine should receive PCV13 first, followed at least one year later by PPSV23. A shorter interval between doses (PCV13 followed ≥8 weeks later by PPSV23) is recommended by the ACIP for adults with immunocompromising conditions and may be appropriate for some travelers with upcoming trips.[1,32]

POLIO — In 2018, the only countries with wild poliovirus circulation during the last 12 months were Pakistan and Afghanistan. Outbreaks of vaccine-derived poliovirus have occurred in some other countries, mainly in Africa.

Recommendations – All persons traveling to countries with wild or vaccine-derived poliovirus circulation should complete a primary series of inactivated polio vaccine (IPV; *Ipol*) before leaving the US. Adults who have not previously been immunized against polio should receive a 3-dose primary series of IPV (2 doses 4-8 weeks apart; third dose 6-12 months after the second). If protection is needed sooner, 2 or 3 doses can be given ≥4 weeks apart; if <4 weeks are available before protection is needed, a single dose is recommended. Adults who previously completed a primary series and have never had a booster should receive a single booster dose of IPV. Previously unimmunized children should receive a 4-dose primary series of IPV beginning at age ≥6 weeks; the first 3 doses should be given ≥4 weeks apart, followed by a fourth dose ≥6 months after the third. A child who received 4 doses before age 4 should be given a fifth dose at age 4-6 years.

Travelers planning to stay for >4 weeks in a country with recent wild or vaccine-derived poliovirus circulation may be required to present proof of polio vaccination when departing that country. Polio vaccination of travelers should be documented on an International Certificate of Vaccination or Prophylaxis (ICVP; "yellow card"). Children and adults who will be in a polio-infected country for >4 weeks, and whose last dose of polio vaccine was administered >12 months before the date they will be leaving that country, should receive an additional dose of IPV before leaving the US. Those who plan to reside in a polio-infected country for >12 months may be required to receive a dose of the polio vaccine that is available in that country (either IPV or oral polio vaccine) between 4 weeks and 12 months before their departure from the polio-infected country.[33]

RABIES — Rabies is highly endemic in many parts of Africa, Asia (particularly India, Pakistan, Bangladesh, and Bali, Indonesia), and Central and South America, but the risk to travelers is generally low.[34]

Recommendations – Pre-exposure vaccination (PrEP) against rabies is recommended for travelers with an occupational risk of exposure, for those (especially children) visiting endemic areas where immediate access to medical treatment, particularly rabies immune globulin (RIG), tends to be limited, and for outdoor-adventure travelers.[35]

After exposure to a potentially rabid animal, persons who received PrEP should promptly receive 2 additional doses of vaccine 3 days apart. For those who did not receive PrEP, the ACIP recommends human RIG plus 4 doses of vaccine given over 14 days; immunosuppressed patients should receive 5 doses of vaccine over 28 days.[36] In one retrospective study, some patients did not develop adequate antibody levels after 4 doses of vaccine.[37]

The Vaccines – Two rabies antigen vaccines are available in the US *(Imovax; RabAvert)*. According to the CDC, cell culture rabies vaccines available outside the US are acceptable alternatives to FDA-approved vaccines, but neural tissue vaccines, which have high rates of serious adverse effects, are not. RIG is not readily available in developing countries, and even when it is, its purity and potency may be less reliable. Purified equine-derived RIG is available in some developing countries and has been used effectively, with a low incidence of adverse effects.

TETANUS, DIPHTHERIA, AND PERTUSSIS — Vaccination against tetanus, diphtheria, and pertussis, which is part of routine childhood immunization in the US, is recommended for all travelers.

Recommendations – Previously unimmunized children should receive 3 or (preferably) 4 doses of pediatric diphtheria, tetanus, and acellular pertussis vaccine (DTaP) before travel. An accelerated schedule can be used beginning at age ≥6 weeks: the first 3 doses are given 4 weeks apart and the fourth dose is given at age ≥12 months and ≥6 months after the third.

Adults with an uncertain history of primary vaccination should receive 3 doses of an inactivated tetanus and diphtheria toxoid (Td) vaccine. The first 2 doses should be administered ≥4 weeks apart and the third 6-12 months after the second. One of the 3 doses (preferably the first) should contain protein components of acellular pertussis combined with diphtheria and tetanus toxoids (Tdap) to also provide protection against pertussis. Two Tdap vaccines *(Adacel; Boostrix)* are available for use in adults, including those ≥65 years old.[38]

A booster dose of inactivated Td vaccine is recommended every 10 years for adults. All persons ≥11 years old who have completed a primary childhood series and have not yet received Tdap vaccine should receive a single dose, which can be given regardless of the interval since the last Td dose to provide pertussis protection before travel. Pregnant women should receive Tdap during each pregnancy.

Tetanus and diphtheria-containing vaccines may interact with carrier proteins on conjugate vaccines, suppressing the immune response to these vaccines; Tdap administration should be deferred until after administration of a meningococcal or pneumococcal conjugate vaccine.[39]

TYPHOID — Typhoid fever is usually acquired through consumption of food or water contaminated with *Salmonella typhi*. The risk is highest in South Asia. Other risk areas are East and Southeast Asia, Central and South America, the Caribbean, and Africa.

Recommendations – Vaccination is recommended for travelers going to areas where there is an increased risk of typhoid fever, especially if they expect a long stay or will be visiting friends or relatives or traveling outside routine tourist destinations.[40,41]

The Vaccines – A live-attenuated oral typhoid vaccine *(Vivotif)* is available for adults and children ≥6 years old. It is taken every other day as a single capsule (at least 1 hour before eating) for a total of 4 doses, beginning at least 2 weeks before departure. The capsules must be refrigerated. Antibiotics should be avoided for at least 24 hours before administration of the first dose and for 1 week after administration of the last dose. The vaccine provides protection for about 5 years.

A purified capsular polysaccharide parenteral vaccine *(Typhim Vi)* is FDA-licensed for use in adults and children ≥2 years old. It is given at least 2 weeks before departure and provides protection for about 2 years. A combined hepatitis A/typhoid vaccine *(Vivaxim)* is available in Canada.

VARICELLA — Varicella is endemic worldwide. Vaccination against varicella has been part of routine childhood immunization in the US since 1996.

Recommendations – Persons born in the US before 1980 are generally considered immune to varicella.[1] Vaccination is recommended for all travelers ≥12 months old without evidence of immunity. Before traveling abroad, children 1-3 years old should receive 1 dose of vaccine and persons ≥4 years old should receive 2 doses. The minimum interval between doses should be 3 months for persons <13 years old and 4 weeks for those ≥13 years old.[28]

The Vaccines – Two varicella-containing vaccines are available in the US: single-antigen varicella vaccine *(Varivax)*, which is licensed for use in persons ≥12 months old, and combination measles-mumps-rubella-varicella vaccine (MMRV; *ProQuad*), which is only licensed for use in children 12 months-12 years old.

YELLOW FEVER — Yellow fever virus is transmitted by the bite of an infected mosquito. It is endemic in tropical South America and sub-Saharan Africa.

Recommendations – The ACIP recommends administration of a single dose of yellow fever vaccine at least 10 days before travel to endemic areas.[42] Booster doses are no longer recommended for most travelers because a single dose has been shown to provide protection for many decades. Additional doses are still recommended for certain populations: women who were pregnant when they received their initial dose should receive one additional dose before traveling to an endemic area; persons who underwent a hematopoietic stem cell transplantation after being vaccinated should be revaccinated before traveling if they are sufficiently immunocompetent; persons who were infected with HIV when they received their last dose should receive a booster dose every 10 years if they continue to be at risk. A booster dose given at least 10 years after the previous dose may also be considered for travelers at increased risk of exposure, such as those planning prolonged travel in an endemic area or those traveling to highly endemic areas during peak transmission season or to an area with an ongoing outbreak.[43]

Some countries require an International Certificate of Vaccination or Prophylaxis (ICVP, "yellow card") as proof of vaccination against yellow fever, or a physician's waiver letter, from all entering travelers; other countries require evidence of vaccination from travelers coming from or traveling through endemic or infected areas, including brief airport transits. An updated list of countries requiring proof of yellow fever vaccination is available at www.cdc.gov/travel.

The Vaccine – US-licensed yellow fever vaccine *(YF-Vax)* is a live-attenuated vaccine prepared in eggs. It is usually available from providers certified by state health departments, but at press time it is temporarily out of stock; supplies are expected to be available by the middle of 2019. Some clinics are offering an alternative IV single-dose live vaccine (*Stamaril* – Sanofi Pasteur). A list of these clinics is available at wwwnc.cdc.gov/travel/page/search-for-stamaril-clinics. *Stamaril*, which has been used for decades in Europe, is available in the US under an investigational new drug program. It is comparable in efficacy and safety to *YF-Vax*.

Yellow fever vaccine-associated viscerotropic disease, a severe systemic illness that can cause fatal organ failure, has been reported rarely. It has occurred only in first-time recipients and is most common in persons >60 years old. Vaccine-associated neurologic disease (encephalitis, Guillain-Barré syndrome, Bell's palsy) has also occurred almost exclusively in first-time recipients; the risk is increased in infants and persons >60 years old.[44,45]

Caution is advised for vaccination of infants 6-8 months old, first-time recipients ≥60 years old, and those with asymptomatic HIV infection and moderate immune suppression (CD4 counts 200-499 cells/mm^3). In a small study, relapse rates were significantly higher among travelers with multiple sclerosis who received yellow fever vaccine.[46] There have been case reports of vaccine-associated neurologic disease in breastfed infants of recently vaccinated women.[47] The vaccine is contraindicated in infants <6 months old, in persons with immunodeficiencies or receiving immunosuppressive or immunomodulatory therapies, and in those with HIV infection and CD4 counts <200 cells/mm[3].[42]

1. Adult immunization. Med Lett Drugs Ther 2018; 60:73.
2. DO Freedman et al. Medical considerations before international travel. N Engl J Med 2016; 375:247.
3. AT Kroger et al. General best practice guidelines for immunization. Best practices guidance of the Advisory Committee on Immunization Practices (ACIP). Available at: https://www.cdc.gov/vaccines/hcp/acip-recs/general-recs/index.html. Accessed November 8, 2018.
4. KK Wong et al. Recommendations of the Advisory Committee on Immunization Practices for use of cholera vaccine. MMWR Morb Mortal Wkly Rep 2017; 66:482.
5. An oral cholera vaccine for travelers (Vaxchora). Med Lett Drugs Ther 2016; 58:113.
6. WH Chen et al. Single-dose live oral cholera vaccine CVD 103-HgR protects against human experimental infection with *Vibrio cholerae* 01 El Tor. Clin Infect Dis 2016; 62:1329.
7. KH Jacobsen. Globalization and the changing epidemiology of hepatitis A virus. Cold Spring Harb Perspect Med 2018; 8(10).
8. A Rosdahl et al. An extra priming dose of hepatitis A vaccine to adult patients with rheumatoid arthritis and drug induced immunosuppression – a prospective, open-label, multi-center study. Travel Med Infect Dis 2018; 21:43.
9. JJ Ott and ST Wiersma. Single-dose administration of inactivated hepatitis A vaccination in the context of hepatitis A vaccine recommendations. Int J Infect Dis 2013; 17:e939.
10. Centers for Disease Control and Prevention. Advisory Committee on Immunization Practices (ACIP) summary report, February 21-22, 2018, Atlanta, Georgia. Available at: www.cdc.gov/vaccines/acip/meetings/downloads/min-archive/min-2018-02-508.pdf. Accessed November 8, 2018.
11. NP Nelson. Updated dosing instructions for immune globulin (human) GamaSTAN S/D for hepatitis A virus prophylaxis. MMWR Morb Mortal Wkly Rep 2017; 66:959.
12. A Schweitzer et al. Estimations of worldwide prevalence of chronic hepatitis B virus infection: a systematic review of data published between 1965 and 2013. Lancet 2015; 386:1546.
13. DF Johnson et al. Hepatitis B and C infection in international travelers. J Travel Med 2013; 20:194.
14. A two-dose hepatitis B vaccine for adults (Heplisav-B). Med Lett Drugs Ther 2018; 60:17.
15. S Schillie et al. Prevention of hepatitis B virus infection in the United States: recommendations of the Advisory Committee on Immunization Practices. MMWR Recomm Rep 2018; 67(1):1.
16. M Goeijenbier et al. Travellers and influenza: risks and prevention. J Travel Med 2016; 24(1).
17. Influenza vaccine for 2018-2019. Med Lett Drugs Ther 2018; 60:169.

18. Centers for Disease Control and Prevention. Use of northern hemisphere influenza vaccines by travelers to the southern hemisphere. MMWR Morb Mortal Wkly Rep 2009; 58:312.
19. SL Hills et al. Japanese encephalitis in travelers from non-endemic countries, 1973-2008. Am J Trop Med Hyg 2010; 82:930.
20. E Mirzaian et al. Mosquito-borne illnesses in travelers: a review of risk and prevention. Pharmacotherapy 2010; 30:1031.
21. A new Japanese encephalitis vaccine (Ixiaro). Med Lett Drugs Ther 2009; 51:66.
22. Use of Japanese encephalitis vaccine in children: recommendations of the advisory committee on immunization practices, 2013. MMWR Morb Mortal Wkly Rep 2013; 62:898.
23. T Jelinek et al. Short-term immunogenicity and safety of an accelerated pre-exposure prophylaxis regimen with Japanese encephalitis vaccine in combination with a rabies vaccine: a phase III multicenter, observer-blind study. J Travel Med 2015; 22:225.
24. JP Cramer et al. One-year immunogenicity kinetics and safety of a purified chick embryo cell rabies vaccine and an inactivated Vero cell-derived Japanese encephalitis vaccine administered concomitantly according to a new, 1-week, accelerated primary series. J Travel Med 2016; 23(3).
25. M Paulke-Korinek et al. Persistence of antibodies six years after booster vaccination with inactivated vaccine against Japanese encephalitis. Vaccine 2015; 33:3600.
26. PA Gastañaduy et al. Measles - United States, January 1-May 23, 2014. MMWR Morbid Mortal Wkly Rep 2014; 63:496.
27. HQ McLean et al. Prevention of measles, rubella, congenital rubella syndrome, and mumps, 2013: summary recommendations of the Advisory Committee on Immunization Practices (ACIP). MMWR Recomm Rep 2013; 62(RR-4):1.
28. Centers for Disease Control and Prevention. CDC Yellow Book 2018: Health Information for International Travel. New York: Oxford University Press, 2017. Available at: https://wwwnc.cdc.gov/travel/page/yellowbook-home. Accessed November 8, 2018.
29. A new conjugate meningococcal vaccine (Menveo). Med Lett Drugs Ther 2010; 52:59.
30. JR MacNeil et al. Use of MenACWY-CRM vaccine in children aged 2 through 23 months at increased risk for meningococcal disease: recommendations of the Advisory Committee on Immunization Practices, 2013. MMWR Morb Mortal Wkly Rep 2014; 63:527.
31. AC Cohn et al. Prevention and control of meningococcal disease: recommendations of the Advisory Committee on Immunization Practices (ACIP). MMWR Recomm Rep 2013; 62(RR-2):1.
32. M Kobayashi et al. Intervals between PCV13 and PPSV23 vaccines: recommendations of the Advisory Committee on Immunization Practices (ACIP). MMWR Morb Mortal Wkly Rep 2015; 64:944.
33. GS Wallace et al. Interim CDC guidance for polio vaccination for travel to and from countries affected by wild poliovirus. MMWR Morb Mortal Wkly Rep 2014; 63:591.
34. C Malerczyk et al. Imported human rabies cases in Europe, the United States, and Japan, 1990 to 2010. J Travel Med 2011; 18:402.
35. AJ Nigg and PL Walker. Overview, prevention, and treatment of rabies. Pharmacotherapy 2009; 29:1182.

36. CE Rupprecht et al. Use of a reduced (4-dose) vaccine schedule for postexposure prophylaxis to prevent human rabies: recommendations of the Advisory Committee on Immunization Practices. MMWR Recomm Rep 2010; 59(RR-2):1.

37. M Uwanyiligira et al. Rabies postexposure prophylaxis in routine practice in view of the new Centers for Disease Control and Prevention and World Health Organization recommendations. Clin Infect Dis 2012; 55:201.

38. Prevention and treatment of pertussis. Med Lett Drugs Ther 2012; 54:73.

39. M Tashani et al. Tetanus-diphtheria-pertussis vaccine may suppress the immune response to subsequent immunization with pneumococcal CRM197-conjugate vaccine (coadministered with quadrivalent meningococcal TT-conjugate vaccine): a randomized, controlled trial. J Travel Med 2017; 24(4).

40. C Greenaway et al. Summary of the Statement on International Travellers and Typhoid by the Committee to Advise on Tropical Medicine and Travel (CATMAT). Can Commun Dis Rep 2014; 40:60.

41. JA Whitaker et al. Rethinking typhoid fever vaccines: implications for travelers and people living in highly endemic areas. J Travel Med 2009; 16:46.

42. JE Staples et al. Yellow fever vaccine: recommendations of the Advisory Committee on Immunization Practices (ACIP). MMWR Recomm Rep 2010; 59(RR-7):1.

43. JE Staples et al. Yellow fever vaccine booster doses: recommendations of the Advisory Committee on Immunization Practices, 2015. MMWR Morb Mortal Wkly Rep 2015; 64:647.

44. RE Thomas et al. How many published cases of serious adverse events after yellow fever vaccination meet Brighton Collaboration diagnostic criteria? Vaccine 2013; 31:6201.

45. RE Thomas et al. The safety of yellow fever vaccine 17D or 17DD in children, pregnant women, HIV+ individuals, and older persons: systematic review. Am J Trop Med Hyg 2012; 86:359.

46. MF Farez and J Correale. Yellow fever vaccination and increased relapse rate in travelers with multiple sclerosis. Arch Neurol 2011; 68:1267.

47. S Kuhn et al. Case report: probable transmission of vaccine strain of yellow fever virus to an infant via breast milk. CMAJ 2011; 183:E243.

ANTIVIRAL DRUGS FOR
Varicella-Zoster Virus and
Herpes Simplex Virus Infections

Original publication date – September 2018

The recommendations for treatment of varicella-zoster virus (VZV) and herpes simplex virus (HSV) infections are listed in tables 1 and 2. Vaccination against VZV was reviewed in a previous issue.[1]

ACYCLOVIR — Acyclovir (*Zovirax*, and generics) is available in topical, oral, and IV formulations. Unlike famciclovir and valacyclovir, acyclovir has poor oral bioavailability; frequent high doses are needed for adequate antiviral activity.

VZV Infection – Oral acyclovir started within 24 hours of rash onset decreases the severity of primary varicella infection (chicken pox).[2]

In patients with localized herpes zoster (latent VZV reactivation), oral acyclovir started within 72 hours of rash onset reduces viral shedding, shortens the duration of rash, and reduces pain severity and duration[3,4]; whether it prevents postherpetic neuralgia is unclear.[5]

IV acyclovir is the treatment of choice for varicella or herpes zoster in patients with severe or disseminated disease. It is also preferred for treatment of severely immunocompromised patients.

Table 1. Drugs for Varicella-Zoster Virus Infection[1]		
Drug[2]	**Usual Adult Dosage[3]**	**Cost[4]**
Primary Varicella Infection (Chicken Pox)[5,6]		
Acyclovir	800 mg PO qid x 5 days	$6.00
or Valacyclovir[7]	1 g PO tid x 5 days	19.50
Herpes Zoster[6,8]		
Acyclovir	800 mg PO 5x/day x 7 days	10.50
or Famciclovir	500 mg PO tid x 7 days	77.90
or Valacyclovir	1 g PO tid x 7 days	27.30
Severe or Disseminated Herpes Zoster		
Acyclovir	10 mg/kg IV q8h x 7 days[9]	137.30
Varicella or Herpes Zoster in Severely Immunocompromised Patients[10]		
Acyclovir	10 mg/kg IV q8h x 7 days[9]	137.30

1. Some of the indications and/or dosages have not been approved by the FDA.
2. Acyclovir and valacyclovir are available as *Zovirax* and *Valtrex*, respectively. Famciclovir is only available generically.
3. Dosage adjustment may be needed for renal or hepatic impairment.
4. Approximate WAC for treatment of a 70-kg patient with the generic product. WAC = wholesaler acquisition cost or manufacturer's published price to wholesalers; WAC represents a published catalogue or list price and may not represent an actual transactional price. Source: AnalySource® Monthly. September 5, 2018. Reprinted with permission by First Databank, Inc. All rights reserved. ©2018. www.fdbhealth.com/policies/drug-pricing-policy.
5. Treatment is effective if started within 24 hours of rash onset. Treatment can be considered for adults and children >12 years old, those with chronic skin or respiratory disorders, those taking a salicylate long term or a corticosteroid, or secondary cases within a household. Antiviral treatment is not recommended for healthy children ≤12 years old with uncomplicated varicella infection.
6. Compared to famciclovir and valacyclovir, acyclovir has poor oral bioavailability; frequent high doses are needed for adequate antiviral activity.
7. Clinical trial data are lacking.
8. Antiviral treatment is recommended for patients ≥50 years old and for those who are immunocompromised or have moderate or severe pain, severe rash, face or eye involvement, or other complications of herpes zoster (J Cohen. N Eng J Med 2013; 369:255).
9. If IV acyclovir is unavailable or VZV is resistant to acyclovir, alternatives include IV ganciclovir and IV foscarnet. Data on their efficacy for this indication are lacking and both drugs are more toxic than IV acyclovir.
10. Includes hematopoietic cell transplant recipients within 4 months of transplantation or with graft-versus-host disease (GVHD) or any transplant patient taking aggressive antirejection medication. For less severely immunocompromised patients with uncomplicated zoster, including most patients with HIV infection, oral valacyclovir or famciclovir can be used.

Suppressive treatment with oral acyclovir is often used to prevent VZV reactivation in immunocompromised patients, including those who have undergone hematopoietic cell transplantation.

HSV Infection – In patients with a first episode of genital herpes (those without prior HSV-1 or -2 infection), oral acyclovir started within 6 days of lesion onset decreases the duration of pain and constitutional symptoms, viral shedding, healing time, and new lesion formation.

Topical acyclovir cream applied 5 times daily reduces the duration of recurrent orolabial herpes by only about 12 hours. In patients with recurrences of orolabial or genital herpes, self-administration of oral acyclovir within 24 hours of symptom onset has been shown to decrease healing time, new lesion formation, and viral shedding by about 1 to 2 days.

Suppressive treatment with oral acyclovir reduces asymptomatic viral shedding, the frequency and severity of symptomatic genital HSV recurrences, and the risk of HSV transmission.[6]

IV acyclovir is the treatment of choice for HSV infections that are visceral, disseminated, or involve the central nervous system (CNS). In neonates with HSV infection, treatment of CNS or disseminated disease with IV acyclovir for a minimum of 3 weeks (2 weeks for localized skin, eye, and mouth disease) reduces morbidity and mortality; 6 months of suppressive treatment with oral acyclovir following acute treatment improves neurodevelopmental outcomes. In the event of an IV acyclovir shortage, the American Academy of Pediatrics recommends IV ganciclovir (first) or IV foscarnet (second) as alternatives; both of these drugs are more toxic than IV acyclovir.[7]

Suppressive treatment with oral acyclovir is often used to prevent HSV reactivation in immunocompromised patients, including hematopoietic cell transplant recipients.

Adverse Effects – Acyclovir is generally well tolerated. GI disturbances, headache, and malaise can occur with systemic administration. Phlebitis and inflammation at the infusion site and reversible renal impairment due to crystalline nephropathy can occur with IV acyclovir; high dosage, rapid infusion, dehydration, and pre-existing renal impairment increase the risk of nephrotoxicity. IV and, rarely, oral acyclovir have been associated with myalgia, rash, Stevens-Johnson syndrome, tremors,

Table 2. Drugs for Herpes Simplex Virus Infections[1]

		Drug[2]
Orolabial		
First episode[5]		Acyclovir
	or	Famciclovir
	or	Valacyclovir
Recurrences[6] –		
Topical[7]		Acyclovir
	or	Docosanol[9]
	or	Penciclovir
Oral		Acyclovir
	or	Famciclovir
	or	Valacyclovir
Suppression[11]		Acyclovir
	or	Famciclovir
	or	Valacyclovir
Genital		
First episode[6]		Acyclovir
	or	Famciclovir
	or	Valacyclovir
Recurrences[6]		Acyclovir
	or	Famciclovir
	or	Valacyclovir

1. Some of the indications and/or dosages have not been approved by the FDA.
2. Acyclovir and valacyclovir are available as *Zovirax* and *Valtrex*, respectively. Famciclovir is only available generically. Penciclovir is available as *Denavir*, docosanol as *Abreva*, trifluridine ophthalmic solution as *Viroptic*, and ganciclovir ophthalmic gel as *Zirgan*.
3. Dosage adjustment may be required for renal or hepatic impairment.
4. Approximate WAC for treatment of a 70-kg patient with the generic product using the lowest dose and shortest treatment duration. Cost of suppressive therapy is for 12 months. WAC = wholesaler acquisition cost or manufacturer's published price to wholesalers; WAC represents a published catalogue or list price and may not represent an actual transactional price. Source: AnalySource® Monthly. September 5, 2018. Reprinted with permission by First Databank, Inc. All rights reserved. ©2018. www.fdbhealth.com/policies/drug-pricing-policy.
5. For moderate or severe primary infection. Clinical trial data establishing the efficacy of recommended drugs and doses are lacking. Some expert clinicians would treat a first episode of orolabial herpes with the same doses used to treat a first episode of genital herpes.
6. Antiviral therapy is most effective when started early.

Usual Adult Dosage[3]	Cost[4]
400 mg PO tid x 7-10 days	$11.90
500 mg PO bid-tid x 7-10 days	52.00
1 g PO bid x 7-10 days	18.20
5% cream 5x/day x 4 days	797.00[8]
10% cream 5x/day until healed (max 10 days)	14.50[8]
1% cream q2h while awake x 4 days	812.00[8]
400 mg PO 5x/day x 5 days	14.00
1500 mg PO single dose[10]	11.10
2 g PO bid x 1 day	5.20
400 mg PO bid[12]	408.80
500 mg PO bid	2708.30
500 mg-1 g PO once/day[13]	297.10
400 mg PO tid x 7-10 days	11.90
or 200 mg 5x/day x 7-10 days[14]	
250 mg PO tid x 7-10 days[14]	34.80
1 g PO bid x 7-10 days[14]	18.20
800 mg PO tid x 2 days or bid x 5 days	8.40
or 400 mg tid x 5 days	
1 g PO bid x 1 day[10]	14.80
or 500 mg x 1 dose, then 250 mg bid x 2 days	
or 125 mg bid x 5 days	
500 mg PO bid x 3 days or 1 g once/d x 5 days	4.90

7. Efficacy is limited. Immunocompromised patients and those with mucosal or disseminated disease should not be treated with topical antiviral drugs.
8. Cost for the smallest available size of the brand name product (acyclovir – *Zovirax*, docosanol – *Abreva*, penciclovir – *Denavir*, trifluridine – *Viroptic*, and ganciclovir – *Zirgan*).
9. Available without a prescription.
10. 500 mg bid x 7 days for patients with HIV infection.
11. Continuous suppressive therapy is recommended for patients with ≥6 recurrent episodes per year and/or severely symptomatic disease. It appears to be safe and has not been associated with emergence of resistance, but some expert clinicians discontinue suppressive treatment for 1-2 months once a year to assess the frequency of recurrences, unless it is being used to reduce the risk of sexual transmission.
12. 400-800 mg bid for patients with HIV infection.
13. 500 mg bid for patients with HIV infection.
14. Treatment can be extended if healing is incomplete after 10 days of therapy.

Continued on next page

Table 2. Drugs for Herpes Simplex Virus Infections[1] (continued)	
	Drug[2]
Genital (continued)	
Suppression[11]	Acyclovir
or	Famciclovir
or	Valacyclovir
Mucocutaneous in Immunocompromised Patients	
	Acyclovir
or	Famciclovir
or	Valacyclovir
Encephalitis	
	Acyclovir[18]
Other Severe or Disseminated Disease	
	Acyclovir[18]
Keratitis[19]	
	Ganciclovir 0.15% ophth gel
or	Trifluridine 1% ophth solution

15. For pregnant women (beginning at 36 weeks gestation), the dose is 400 mg tid.
16. 500 mg once/day for immunocompetent patients with <10 recurrences per year and 500 mg bid or 1 g/day for patients with ≥10 recurrences per year.
17. For pregnant women (beginning at 36 weeks gestation), the dose is 500 mg bid.
18. If IV acyclovir is unavailable or HSV is resistant to acyclovir, alternatives include IV ganciclovir and IV foscarnet. Data on their efficacy in treating herpes encephalitis are lacking and both drugs are more toxic than IV acyclovir. Oral valacyclovir may achieve therapeutic levels in the CSF (T Pouplin et al. Antimicrob Agent Chemother 2011; 55:3624), but its use is not generally recommended because of the severity of the disease and the uncertainty of adequate GI absorption.

lethargy, confusion, hallucinations, seizures, encephalopathy, and coma. CNS adverse effects are more likely to occur in older patients and in those with renal impairment. Neutropenia and other hematologic toxicities have been reported rarely. Application-site reactions can occur with topical acyclovir.

Pregnancy and Lactation – Use of acyclovir during pregnancy has not been associated with an increased risk of congenital anomalies.[8] Many expert clinicians prefer acyclovir over famciclovir or valacyclovir in

Usual Adult Dosage[3]	Cost[4]
400 mg PO bid[12,15]	$408.80
250 mg PO bid[13]	1209.60
500 mg-1 g PO once/day[13,16,17]	297.10
5 mg/kg IV q8h x 7-14 days	73.20
or 400 mg PO 5x/day x 7-10 days	
500 mg PO bid x 7-10 days	52.00
500 mg-1 g PO bid x 7-10 days	11.40
10-15 mg/kg IV q8h x 14-21 days	274.50
5-10 mg/kg IV q8h x 14-21 days	146.40
1 drop q3h while awake[20]	331.40[8]
1 drop q2h while awake (max 9 drops/day)[20]	372.90[8]

19. An ophthalmic preparation of acyclovir is available in some countries. Treatment of HSV ocular infection should be supervised by an ophthalmologist; duration of therapy and dosage depend on response. Oral antivirals (acyclovir, valacyclovir, famciclovir) are probably as effective as ophthalmic preparations without adverse ocular effects.
20. Once the cornea has re-epithelialized, the dosage can be decreased to 1 drop q4h while awake x 7 days for trifluridine and 1 drop tid x 7 days for ganciclovir.

pregnant women because of extensive experience with its use during pregnancy. Acyclovir is excreted in human breast milk following systemic administration.

The American College of Obstetricians and Gynecologists recommends offering suppressive acyclovir therapy (400 mg three times daily beginning at week 36) to pregnant women with active recurrent genital herpes to reduce the risk of recurrence at delivery and possibly the need for cesarean section.[9] Suppressive treatment reduces, but does not eliminate, viral shedding; maternal-fetal transmission of HSV infection has been reported in some women taking acyclovir suppressive therapy.

Resistance – Despite widespread use, VZV and HSV resistance to acyclovir rarely develops in immunocompetent patients (prevalence <1%). Almost all acyclovir-resistant HSV infections have occurred in immunocompromised patients treated with the drug; these isolates are usually cross-resistant to famciclovir. Valacyclovir is a prodrug of acyclovir; isolates resistant to acyclovir are also resistant to valacyclovir. Acyclovir-resistant VZV or HSV infections may respond to IV foscarnet.

VALACYCLOVIR — Valacyclovir (*Valtrex*, and generics) is metabolized to acyclovir after oral administration, resulting in a 3- to 5-fold increase in bioavailability compared to oral acyclovir.

VZV Infection – Valacyclovir 1 gram three times daily is at least as effective as acyclovir 800 mg 5 times daily in decreasing healing time and pain duration in patients with localized herpes zoster. Oral valacyclovir has been effective for treatment of uncomplicated herpes zoster in immunocompromised patients, but data on its use in severely immunocompromised patients are lacking.

Suppressive treatment with valacyclovir has reduced VZV reactivation in hematopoietic cell transplant recipients.[10]

HSV Infection – For episodic treatment of orolabial herpes, oral valacyclovir 2 grams twice daily for one day reduced healing time by about 1 day.[11] In first-episode or recurrent genital herpes, valacyclovir given twice daily for 7-10 days is as effective as acyclovir given 5 times daily for 7-10 days.

Valacyclovir 500 mg once daily is effective for suppression of recurrent genital herpes; a higher dose may be needed for patients with frequent recurrences (≥10 per year). Valacyclovir has been shown to be more effective than famciclovir for this indication.[12]

In HSV-discordant heterosexual couples, suppressive treatment of the infected partner with once-daily valacyclovir can reduce the risk of HSV transmission by about 50%.[13] Suppressive treatment can also reduce the risk of transmission when used by persons who have multiple partners (including men who have sex with men) and by those who are HSV-2 seropositive without a history of genital herpes.[14]

Adverse Effects – Valacyclovir is generally well tolerated; adverse effects are similar to those with acyclovir. Thrombotic thrombocytopenic purpura and hemolytic uremic syndrome have been reported in some severely immunocompromised patients taking high doses of valacyclovir (8 grams/day).

Pregnancy and Lactation – As with acyclovir, use of valacyclovir during pregnancy has not been associated with an increased risk of major birth defects.[8] However, many expert clinicians prefer acyclovir over famciclovir or valacyclovir in pregnant women because of extensive experience with its use during pregnancy. Acyclovir is excreted in breast milk following ingestion of oral valacyclovir.

Resistance – Valacyclovir is a prodrug of acyclovir; isolates resistant to acyclovir are also resistant to valacyclovir. IV foscarnet may be effective against valacyclovir-resistant strains.

FAMCICLOVIR — Famciclovir is rapidly converted to penciclovir after oral administration.

VZV Infection – In patients with herpes zoster, famciclovir started within 48 hours of rash onset decreases healing time and pain duration.

HSV Infection – Famciclovir is effective for treatment of first episodes and recurrences of genital HSV infection and for chronic suppression. Single-day, patient-initiated famciclovir treatment has been shown to reduce healing time of recurrent orolabial herpes and genital herpes lesions by 1-2 days compared to placebo.[15,16] It is similar in efficacy and safety to a 3-day course of valacyclovir for treatment of recurrent genital herpes.[17] Valacyclovir has been shown to be more effective than famciclovir for suppression of recurrent genital herpes and reduction of viral shedding.[12]

Adverse Effects – Famciclovir is generally well tolerated. Headache, nausea, and diarrhea can occur. Thrombocytopenia, confusion, hallucinations, and nephrotoxicity have been reported.

Pregnancy and Lactation – As with acyclovir, use of famciclovir during pregnancy has not been associated with an increased risk of major birth defects.[8] However, many expert clinicians prefer acyclovir over famciclovir or valacyclovir in pregnant women because of extensive experience with its use during pregnancy. Whether famciclovir or penciclovir is excreted in human breast milk is unknown. Penciclovir is excreted in rat milk at concentrations higher than those in plasma.

Resistance – Acyclovir-resistant HSV and VZV strains are generally also resistant to famciclovir. IV foscarnet may be effective against famciclovir-resistant strains.

IMMUNE GLOBULIN FOR VZV — Varicella zoster immune globulin (human; *Varizig*) is FDA-approved for postexposure prophylaxis against VZV in persons at high risk for severe disease who lack evidence of immunity to VZV and for whom VZV vaccine is contraindicated. The CDC recommends that one dose of varicella zoster immune globulin be given as soon as possible, but preferably within 10 days, after VZV exposure to pregnant or immunocompromised patients without evidence of immunity, newborn infants whose mothers had signs and symptoms of VZV infection around the time of delivery, and hospitalized premature infants. A second dose of immunoglobulin can be considered for high-risk patients who have additional exposures to VZV >3 weeks after the first dose.[18]

OTHER DRUGS FOR HSV — **Topical** – Penciclovir 1% cream *(Denavir)* and docosanol 10% cream (*Abreva*; available over the counter) are FDA-approved for treatment of orolabial herpes. Like topical acyclovir, they minimally reduce healing time, are applied multiple times per day, and can cause application-site reactions such as rash and pruritus.

Imiquimod cream *(Zyclara, and others)* and cidofovir gel, which must be compounded at a pharmacy, have been used off-label for treatment of acyclovir-resistant genital HSV infection.[19]

In a randomized, double-blind trial, the rate of HSV-2 acquisition in HSV-2-negative women was significantly lower with pericoital application of tenofovir gel (not available in the US) than with placebo (10.2 vs 21.0 cases per 100 person-years).[20]

Ophthalmic – Trifluridine ophthalmic solution (*Viroptic*, and generics), a nucleoside analog active against HSV, including some acyclovir-resistant strains, is FDA-approved for treatment of primary HSV keratoconjunctivitis and recurrent epithelial keratitis. Ganciclovir gel *(Zirgan)* is FDA-approved for treatment of acute herpetic keratitis (dendritic ulcers).

1. Adult immunization. Med Lett Drugs Ther 2018; 60:73.
2. J Cohen and J Breuer. Chickenpox: treatment. BMJ Clin Evid 2015; 2015:0192.
3. JI Cohen. Clinical practice: herpes zoster. N Engl J Med 2013; 369:255.
4. RH Dworkin et al. Recommendations for the management of herpes zoster. Clin Infect Dis 2007; 44:S1.
5. N Chen et al. Antiviral treatment for preventing postherpetic neuralgia. Cochrane Database Syst Rev 2014; 2:CD006866.
6. JW Gnann Jr. and RJ Whitley. Clinical practice: genital herpes. N Engl J Med 2016; 375:666.
7. JB Harris and AP Holmes. Neonatal herpes simplex viral infections and acyclovir: an update. J Pediatr Pharmacol Ther 2017; 22:88.
8. B Pasternak and A Hviid. Use of acyclovir, valacyclovir, and famciclovir in the first trimester of pregnancy and the risk of birth defects. JAMA 2010; 304:859.
9. American College of Obstetricians and Gynecologists Committee on Practice Bulletins. ACOG Practice Bulletin. No. 82 June 2007. Management of herpes in pregnancy. Obstet Gynecol 2007; 109:1489.
10. F Sahoo et al. Herpes zoster in autologous hematopoietic cell transplant recipients in the era of acyclovir or valacyclovir prophylaxis and novel treatment and maintenance therapies. Biol Blood Marrow Transplant 2017; 23:505.
11. SL Spruance et al. High-dose, short-duration, early valacyclovir therapy for episodic treatment of cold sores: results of two randomized, placebo-controlled, multicenter studies. Antimicrob Agents Chemother 2003; 47:1072.

12. A Wald et al. Comparative efficacy of famciclovir and valacyclovir for suppression of recurrent genital herpes and viral shedding. Sex Transm Dis 2006; 33:529.
13. L Corey et al. Once-daily valacyclovir to reduce the risk of transmission of genital herpes. N Engl J Med 2004; 350:11.
14. KA Workowski et al. Sexually transmitted diseases treatment guidelines, 2015. MMWR Recomm Rep 2015; 64:1.
15. SL Spruance et al. Single-dose, patient-initiated famciclovir: a randomized, double-blind, placebo-controlled trial for episodic treatment of herpes labialis. J Am Acad Dermatol 2006; 55:47.
16. FY Aoki et al. Single-day, patient-initiated famciclovir therapy for recurrent genital herpes: a randomized, double-blind, placebo-controlled trial. Clin Infect Dis 2006; 42:8.
17. M Abudalu et al. Single-day, patient-initiated famciclovir therapy versus 3-day valacyclovir regimen for recurrent genital herpes: a randomized, double-blind, comparative trial. Clin Infect Dis 2008; 47:651.
18. CDC. Updated recommendations for use of VariZig – United States, 2013. MMWR Morbid Mortal Wkly Rep 2013; 62:574.
19. N Perkins et al. Topical imiquimod treatment of acyclovir-resistant herpes simplex disease: case series and literature review. Sex Transm Infect 2011; 87:292.
20. SS Abdool Karim et al. Tenofovir gel for the prevention of herpes simplex virus type 2 infection. N Engl J Med 2015; 373:530.

DRUGS FOR TREATMENT AND PREVENTION OF
Venous Thromboembolism

Original publication date – March 2018

Anticoagulants are the drugs of choice for treatment and prevention of deep venous thrombosis (DVT) and pulmonary embolism (PE), collectively referred to as venous thromboembolism (VTE). Updated US guidelines for treatment of VTE were published in 2016.[1,2]

STANDARD TREATMENT — Most patients with acute VTE have traditionally been treated initially (5-10 days) with a parenteral anticoagulant such as low-molecular-weight heparin (LMWH), fondaparinux (*Arixtra*, and generics), or unfractionated heparin (UFH), with an oral vitamin K antagonist such as warfarin (*Coumadin*, and others) started at the same time. After the parenteral anticoagulant is stopped, warfarin is continued for at least 3 months and sometimes indefinitely.[3,4] Two direct oral anticoagulants (DOACs), apixaban *(Eliquis)* and rivaroxaban *(Xarelto)*, have recently been approved as monotherapy for initial treatment of VTE, and two others, dabigatran *(Pradaxa)* and edoxaban *(Savaysa)*, have been approved for use after initial treatment with a parenteral anticoagulant.

For primary prevention of VTE, LMWH has generally been recommended for orthopedic and nonorthopedic surgery patients for whom postoperative prophylaxis is indicated. Rivaroxaban and apixaban

Recommendations
Treatment of Acute VTE
▸ LMWH or fondaparinux, with or without warfarin, has generally been recommended for initial treatment (5-10 days) of acute deep venous thrombosis (DVT) or pulmonary embolism (PE).
▸ Apixaban and rivaroxaban are oral alternatives for initial use as monotherapy in patients without active cancer.
▸ If a parenteral anticoagulant (UFH, LMWH, or fondaparinux) is used for initial treatment, warfarin or a DOAC (apixaban, rivaroxaban, dabigatran, or edoxaban) can be used for long-term treatment. A DOAC is preferred over warfarin.
▸ LMWH is recommended for initial and long-term treatment of patients with active cancer.
▸ Warfarin or UFH is recommended for treatment of patients with CrCl <30 mL/min.
▸ LMWH is recommended for use during pregnancy.
Duration of Anticoagulation
▸ Patients with VTE should be treated for a minimum of 3 months.
▸ Patients with an unprovoked VTE and those with active cancer have the highest risk of recurrence; they should generally be treated for >3 months and sometimes indefinitely.
Extended Treatment
▸ After 6-12 months of anticoagulation therapy, extended treatment for one year with low doses of apixaban or rivaroxaban can prevent symptomatic recurrences of VTE.
▸ After stopping an anticoagulant, aspirin therapy can reduce the risk of recurrence.
Primary Prevention of VTE
▸ LMWH is recommended for prevention of VTE in most orthopedic and nonorthopedic surgical patients for whom postoperative prophylaxis is indicated.
▸ Apixaban, rivaroxaban, and dabigatran are oral alternatives for prevention of VTE in patients undergoing knee or hip replacement surgery.
▸ The DOAC betrixaban is an oral alternative to parenteral treatment in patients hospitalized for an acute medical illness who are at increased risk of thrombosis.

are FDA-approved for prevention of VTE after knee or hip replacement surgery. Dabigatran is approved after hip replacement surgery.

PARENTERAL ANTICOAGULANTS

HEPARIN — Heparins act by combining with plasma antithrombin to form a complex that is more active in neutralizing thrombin and factor Xa than antithrombin alone. UFH has some disadvantages compared to LMWH: it is more likely to cause heparin-induced thrombocytopenia and has a more variable anticoagulant response that requires monitoring. However, UFH also has some advantages over LMWH that have kept it from becoming obsolete: its anticoagulant effect can be rapidly and completely reversed by protamine, it is not renally eliminated and may be safer in patients with renal impairment, and it directly inhibits the contact activation pathway that is important in the formation of thrombi in stents, catheters, and extracorporeal circuits.[5,6] The shorter half-life of UFH may also be advantageous in patients who are at high risk of bleeding.

LMWH — The low-molecular-weight heparins enoxaparin (*Lovenox*, and generics) and dalteparin *(Fragmin)*, which are produced by cleaving UFH into shorter chains, inhibit factor Xa more than they inhibit thrombin. Compared to UFH, LMWH has a longer half-life that permits fewer doses per day. LMWH also binds less to platelets and plasma proteins, which leads to greater bioavailability and a more predictable anticoagulant response. In clinical trials comparing it with UFH, LMWH has generally been at least as safe and as effective for prevention and treatment of VTE. For initial treatment of VTE, LMWH is generally preferred over UFH.

FONDAPARINUX — A synthetic analog of the pentasaccharide sequence of heparin, fondaparinux binds antithrombin with high affinity and indirectly inhibits factor Xa. The drug has a long half-life and requires injection only once daily. Fondaparinux appears to be as effective as UFH or LMWH for prevention and treatment of VTE, and it is much less likely to cause heparin-induced thrombocytopenia. Fondaparinux accumulates in patients with renal impairment; it is contraindicated for use in patients with CrCl <30 mL/min.

Table 1. Some Parenteral Anticoagulants for VTE[1]	
Drug	**Usual Adult Treatment Dosage**
Unfractionated Heparin (UFH)	
generic	80 units/kg IV bolus, then 18 units/kg/hr IV[4] or 333 units/kg SC initially, followed by 250 units/kg SC q12h[4]
Low-Molecular-Weight Heparins (LMWHs)	
Dalteparin − *Fragmin* (Pfizer)	200 IU/kg SC once/d[4,5,6]
Enoxaparin − generic *Lovenox* (Sanofi)	1 mg/kg SC bid or 1.5 mg/kg SC once/d[4,5]
Direct Thrombin Inhibitor	
Desirudin − *Iprivask* (Valeant)	Not an FDA-approved indication
Factor Xa Inhibitor	
Fondaparinux − generic *Arixtra* (Mylan)	5-10 mg SC once/d[4,5,9,10]

1. See Table 3 on pages 240-241 for FDA-approved VTE indications.
2. Prophylaxis is recommended for ≥10-14 days and for up to 35 days after major orthopedic surgery (Y Falck-Ytter et al. Chest 2012; 141:e278S).
3. Approximate WAC for 30 days' treatment of a 70-kg patient at the lowest usual adult dosage for treatment. WAC = wholesaler acquisition cost or manufacturer's published price to wholesalers; WAC represents a published catalogue or list price and may not represent an actual transactional price. Source: AnalySource® Monthly. February 5, 2018. Reprinted with permission by First Databank, Inc. All rights reserved. ©2018. www.fdbhealth.com/policies/drug-pricing-policy.
4. Warfarin is generally started at the same time. The parenteral anticoagulant can be stopped after a minimum of 5 days when INR is ≥2 for at least 24 hours (MA Smythe et al. J Thromb Thrombolysis 2016; 41:165).

DESIRUDIN — The hirudin analog desirudin *(Iprivask)* is a direct thrombin inhibitor. Unlike heparins and fondaparinux, direct thrombin inhibitors inhibit clot-bound as well as circulating thrombin. It appears to be more effective than UFH or LMWH for prevention of VTE, but it must be injected twice daily and can cause life-threatening allergic reactions.

ORAL ANTICOAGULANTS

WARFARIN — Warfarin is effective for prevention and treatment of VTE and does not require dosage adjustments in patients with renal impairment, but it can take up to 7 days to achieve a full therapeutic

Usual Adult Prophylaxis Dosage[2]	Cost[3]
5000 units SC q8-12h	$651.00
2500-5000 IU SC once/d[5]	3527.40
30 mg SC bid or 40 mg SC once/d[5]	630.00
	3473.40
15 mg SC q12h[5,7]	5400.00[8]
2.5 mg SC once/d[5,10,11]	1755.00
	3926.10

5. Dosage adjustments may be needed for renal impairment.
6. For extended VTE treatment in patients with cancer, the dose is 200 IU/kg SC once/d for 30 days, followed by 150 IU/kg SC once/d x 5 months (max 18,000 IU/day).
7. Has only been studied for up to 12 days' use.
8. Cost for 12 days' prophylaxis.
9. Dose is 5 mg if patient weighs <50 kg, 7.5 mg if 50-100 kg, 10 mg if >100 kg.
10. Contraindicated in patients with CrCl <30 mL/min.
11. Dosage for adults weighing >50 kg. Contraindicated in patients weighing <50 kg.

effect. Drawbacks include variability in dosage requirements, dietary restrictions, drug interactions, and the need for close monitoring to keep the INR in the therapeutic range.

DIRECT ORAL ANTICOAGULANTS (DOACs) — Five DOACs are now available in the US (see Table 3). They appear to be effective and safe for prevention and treatment of VTE without INR monitoring in patients without active cancer, but data in older patients and those with renal impairment are limited.[7] DOACs have shorter half-lives than warfarin, which increases the risk of thrombosis with missed doses. Large head-to-head trials of these drugs are lacking.

Table 2. Some Oral Anticoagulants for VTE[1]	
Drug	**Usual Adult Treatment Dosage**
Vitamin K Antagonist	

Warfarin – generic
  Coumadin (BMS)
  Jantoven (USL)
	2-10 mg once/d[4,5]

Direct Thrombin Inhibitor	
Dabigatran etexilate – *Pradaxa* (Boehringer Ingelheim)	150 mg bid[6-9]
Factor Xa Inhibitors	
Apixaban – *Eliquis* (BMS)	10 mg bid x 7 days, then 5 mg bid[10,11]
Betrixaban – *Bevyxxa* (Portola)	Not an FDA-approved indication
Edoxaban – *Savaysa* (Daiichi-Sankyo)	60 mg once/d[6,9,14]
Rivaroxaban – *Xarelto* (Janssen)	15 mg bid x 3 weeks, then 20 mg once/d[6,8,15,16]

1. See Table 3 on pages 240-241 for FDA-approved VTE indications.
2. Prophylaxis is recommended for a minimum of 10-14 days and for up to 35 days after major orthopedic surgery (Y Falck-Ytter et al. Chest 2012; 141:e278S).
3. Approximate WAC for 30 days' treatment at the lowest usual adult dosage for treatment. Cost of betrixaban is based on dosage for prophylaxis. WAC = wholesaler acquisition cost or manufacturer's published price to wholesalers; WAC represents a published catalogue or list price and may not represent an actual transactional price. Source: AnalySource® Monthly. February 5, 2018. Reprinted with permission by First Databank, Inc. All rights reserved. ©2018. www.fdbhealth.com/policies/drug-pricing-policy.
4. Monitor daily and adjust dose until INR is in therapeutic range (INR 2-3).
5. Requires overlap with LMWH, fondaparinux, or UFH for ≥5 days and until INR is ≥2 for at least 24 hours.
6. Dosage adjustments may be needed for renal impairment.
7. Avoid coadministration with P-glycoprotein (P-gp) inhibitors in patients with CrCl <50 mL/min.
8. Should not be used in patients with CrCl <30 mL/min.

Dabigatran – In patients with acute VTE treated initially for 5-10 days with UFH or LMWH, the direct thrombin inhibitor dabigatran was as effective and safe as warfarin in preventing recurrent VTE.[8] For extended treatment of VTE (after 3-12 months of initial treatment), dabigatran was noninferior to warfarin and had a lower risk of major bleeding.[9] Because of multiple reports of severe, sometimes fatal bleeding with dabigatran, the FDA conducted a postmarketing study in >134,000 patients ≥65 years old; it found that the risks of intracranial bleeding and death were lower with dabigatran than with warfarin, but the risk of major GI bleeding was higher with dabigatran.[10]

Usual Adult Prophylaxis Dosage[2]	Cost[3]
2-10 mg once/d[4]	$7.80
	64.50
	10.80
110 mg once, then 220 mg once/d[6-8]	400.60
2.5 mg bid[10]	419.00
160 mg once, then 80 mg once/d for a total of 35-42 d[6,12,13]	450.00
Not an FDA-approved indication	336.60
10 mg once/d[6,8]	333.30

9. FDA-approved for treatment of VTE following 5-10 days of initial therapy with a parenteral anticoagulant.
10. When coadministered with dual strong CYP3A4/P-gp inhibitors, reduce dose by 50%; patients taking 2.5 mg bid should not take dual strong CYP3A4/P-gp inhibitors.
11. For extended treatment after at least 6 months of treatment for DVT or PE, the dosage for reduction in risk of recurrence of VTE is 2.5 mg bid.
12. Should not be used in patients with CrCl <15 mL/min.
13. Dosage in patients taking a P-gp inhibitor concurrently is 80 mg once, then 40 mg once/d.
14. Dosage is 30 mg once/d in patients taking a P-gp inhibitor concurrently or who weigh ≤60 kg.
15. Avoid coadministration with dual P-gp/strong CYP3A4 inhibitors or inducers. Avoid coadministration in patients with CrCl 15-<80 mL/min taking dual P-gp/moderate CYP3A4 inhibitors.
16. For extended treatment after at least 6 months of treatment for DVT or PE, the dosage for reduction in risk of recurrence of VTE is 10 mg once/d.

Rivaroxaban – The direct factor Xa inhibitor rivaroxaban was more effective than enoxaparin in preventing VTE and death after elective hip or knee arthroplasty, but it had a higher risk of major and other clinically relevant bleeding.[11] Rivaroxaban was noninferior to enoxaparin followed by a vitamin K antagonist for treatment of acute VTE, with no increase in major or other clinically relevant bleeding.[12,13]

Apixaban – In two randomized, controlled trials, the direct factor Xa inhibitor apixaban was more effective than enoxaparin in preventing VTE or death after knee or hip replacement, with no increase in major or

Table 3. FDA-Approved Indications of Anticoagulants for VTE
Heparin
Unfractionated Heparin ► Prophylaxis of DVT and PE ► Treatment of DVT and PE
Low Molecular-Weight Heparins (LMWHs)
Enoxaparin (*Lovenox*, and generics) ► Prophylaxis of DVT following abdominal surgery or hip or knee replacement surgery ► Prophylaxis of DVT in medical patients with severely restricted mobility during acute illness ► Treatment of acute DVT (without PE in outpatients and with or without PE in inpatients)
Dalteparin (*Fragmin*) ► Prophylaxis of DVT following abdominal surgery or hip replacement surgery ► Prophylaxis of DVT in medical patients with severely restricted mobility during acute illness ► Reduction in the risk of recurrent symptomatic VTE in cancer patients (extended treatment for 6 months)
Parenteral Direct Thrombin Inhibitor
Desirudin (*Iprivask*) ► Prophylaxis of DVT following hip replacement surgery
Parenteral Factor Xa Inhibitor
Fondaparinux (*Arixtra*, and generics) ► Prophylaxis of DVT following hip fracture surgery, hip or knee replacement surgery, or abdominal surgery ► Treatment of acute DVT or PE in combination with warfarin
Vitamin K Antagonist
Warfarin (*Coumadin*, and others) ► Prophylaxis of DVT and PE ► Treatment of DVT and PE

Continued on next page

other clinically relevant bleeding.[14,15] In a 6-month, randomized, double-blind trial in 5395 patients with acute VTE, apixaban was noninferior to

Table 3. FDA-Approved Indications of Anticoagulants for VTE (continued)
Direct Oral Anticoagulants (DOACs)
Apixaban *(Eliquis)* ▸ Prophylaxis of DVT following hip or knee replacement surgery ▸ Treatment of DVT and PE ▸ Reduction in the risk of recurrent DVT and PE following initial treatment lasting at least 6 months
Betrixaban *(Bevyxxa)* ▸ Prophylaxis of VTE in patients hospitalized for an acute medical illness who are at risk for thromboembolic complications due to moderate or severe restricted mobility and other risk factors for VTE
Dabigatran etexilate *(Pradaxa)* ▸ Prophylaxis of DVT and PE following hip replacement surgery ▸ Treatment of DVT and PE following 5-10 days of initial therapy with a parenteral anticoagulant ▸ Reduction in the risk of recurrent DVT and PE following initial therapy
Edoxaban *(Savaysa)* ▸ Treatment of DVT and PE following 5-10 days of initial therapy with a parenteral anticoagulant
Rivaroxaban *(Xarelto)* ▸ Prophylaxis of DVT following hip or knee replacement surgery ▸ Treatment of DVT and PE ▸ Reduction in the risk of recurrent DVT and/or PE following initial treatment lasting at least 6 months

enoxaparin plus warfarin in preventing recurrent VTE or VTE-related death, and major bleeding occurred less frequently with apixaban (0.6% vs 1.8%).[16]

Edoxaban – In a randomized, double-blind trial in 8240 patients with acute VTE treated initially with UFH or enoxaparin, the once-daily direct factor Xa inhibitor edoxaban was noninferior to warfarin in preventing recurrent VTE or VTE-related death, and patients taking edoxaban had a significantly lower rate of major or clinically relevant nonmajor bleeding (8.5% vs 10.3%).[17]

Betrixaban – The direct factor Xa inhibitor betrixaban *(Bevyxxa)* is approved by the FDA only for prevention of VTE in adults hospitalized for an acute medical illness who have moderately or severely restricted mobility and other risk factors for VTE. In a double-blind trial in 7441 such patients, longer-duration treatment (35-42 days) with once-daily betrixaban was more effective in preventing VTE than shorter-duration treatment (6-14 days) with the LMWH enoxaparin.[18]

CHOICE OF ANTICOAGULANTS — Previous CHEST guidelines have recommended warfarin over LMWH for long-term treatment of VTE in **patients without active cancer**, who generally have low rates of recurrence. Recent studies have shown that DOACs (apixaban, dabigatran, edoxaban, and rivaroxaban) are as effective as warfarin in treating VTE, with a lower risk of intracranial bleeding.[19] Based on these findings and the greater convenience of the DOACs, which do not require INR monitoring, the 2016 guidelines recommend that they be used for long-term treatment of VTE in patients without active cancer. No large trials directly comparing the DOACs have been published. Indirect evidence suggests that apixaban may have the lowest rate of major bleeding.[20] Apixaban and rivaroxaban are oral alternatives to parenteral anticoagulants for initial treatment of VTE.

The 2016 CHEST guidelines recommend LMWH for initial and long-term treatment of VTE in **patients with active cancer**.[1] In a randomized trial in 900 such patients with acute, symptomatic VTE treated initially with the LMWH tinzaparin (no longer available in the US), continued treatment with tinzaparin was not significantly more effective than warfarin in preventing recurrences (6.9% vs 10.0%). There were no differences between the drugs in major bleeding or death, but tinzaparin was associated with a significantly lower risk of clinically relevant nonmajor bleeding than warfarin (10.9% vs 15.3%).[21] In an open-label, randomized trial in 1046 patients with active cancer, the DOAC edoxaban was noninferior to the LMWH dalteparin for treatment of acute VTE. The rate of recurrent VTE was not significantly lower with edoxaban than with

Table 4. Duration of Anticoagulation for VTE[1]

VTE	Recurrence Rate[2]	Bleeding Risk[3]	Duration of Anticoagulation[4]
Provoked by surgery	3%	any	3 months
Not provoked by surgery[5]	15%	any	3 months
Unprovoked	30%	high	3 months
		moderate, low	>3 months
Cancer-associated	15%[6]	any	>3 months

1. C Kearon et al. Chest 2016; 149:315.
2. At 5 years.
3. Patients are considered low, moderate, or high risk based on whether they have 0, 1, or ≥2 risk factors, respectively. Risk factors include age >75 years, previous bleeding, cancer, metastatic cancer, renal failure, hepatic failure, thrombocytopenia, previous stroke, diabetes, anemia, antiplatelet therapy, recent surgery, frequent falls, alcohol abuse, and use of NSAIDs.
4. >3 months means there is no scheduled stop date.
5. Provoked by estrogen therapy, pregnancy, leg injury, or flight >8 hours.
6. Annualized risk of recurrence. Recurrence at 5 years not estimated because of cancer-associated mortality.

dalteparin (7.9% vs 11.3%), but the rate of major bleeding, mainly upper GI bleeding, was significantly higher with edoxaban (6.9% vs 4.0%).[22,23]

For patients with **severe renal impairment** (CrCl <30 mL/min), warfarin or UFH, which do not require dosage adjustments, are recommended for treatment of VTE.

Dabigatran, which has been associated with an increased risk of acute coronary events, is not recommended for VTE treatment in patients with **coronary artery disease**.[24]

Warfarin should not be used in patients with an increased INR at baseline who have **chronic liver disease**, which makes INR monitoring unreliable[25]; LMWH is preferred in such patients.

DURATION OF ANTICOAGULATION — The recommended durations of anticoagulant treatment for VTE in the CHEST guidelines (see Table 4) are based on the risk of recurrence over 5 years in four subgroups of patients and their risk factors for bleeding, which include age >75 years, previous bleeding, cancer, metastatic cancer, renal failure, hepatic failure, thrombocytopenia, previous stroke, diabetes, anemia, antiplatelet therapy, recent surgery, frequent falls, alcohol abuse, and use of NSAIDs. Patients are considered low, moderate, or high risk based on whether they have 0, 1, or ≥2 risk factors, respectively.

EXTENDED TREATMENT — There is a risk of recurrence of VTE when anticoagulants are stopped. To reduce the risk of bleeding, extended treatment with lower-dose anticoagulant therapy or aspirin can be considered.

Aspirin – Two randomized, double-blind trials examined the efficacy and safety of extended treatment with aspirin for a first unprovoked VTE. A double-blind trial in 402 patients who had completed 6 to 18 months of oral anticoagulant treatment compared extended treatment for 2 years with aspirin 100 mg to placebo; the annual VTE recurrence rate was 6.6% in patients who received aspirin 100 mg and 11.2% in those who received placebo, a significant difference, and there was one major bleeding episode in each group.[26] A double-blind, placebo-controlled trial in 822 patients who had completed initial anticoagulant treatment for a first unprovoked VTE compared aspirin 100 mg to placebo for 4 years; the rate of a composite of VTE, MI, stroke, major bleeding, or death was reduced by 33% in patients who received aspirin 100 mg, and there were no significant differences between the two groups in bleeding rates.[27] The recent CHEST guidelines concluded that aspirin is not a reasonable alternative to an anticoagulant for extended treatment of VTE, but aspirin can reduce the rate of recurrence in patients who are no longer taking an anticoagulant.[1]

Apixaban – In a randomized, double-blind, 12-month trial in 2482 patients with VTE who had completed 6-12 months of anticoagulation therapy, a symptomatic recurrence (fatal or nonfatal) occurred in 1.7% of those taking apixaban 2.5 mg (half the usual treatment dose), 1.7% of those taking apixaban 5 mg, and 8.8% of those taking placebo. Rates of major bleeding were 0.2% with apixaban 2.5 mg, 0.1% with apixaban 5 mg, and 0.5% with placebo.[28]

Rivaroxaban – In a randomized, double-blind, 12-month trial in 3365 patients with VTE who had completed 6-12 months of anticoagulation therapy, a symptomatic recurrence (fatal or nonfatal) occurred in 1.2% of patients taking rivaroxaban 10 mg (half the usual treatment dose), 1.5% of those taking rivaroxaban 20 mg, and 4.4% of those taking aspirin 100 mg. Rates of major bleeding were 0.4% with rivaroxaban 10 mg, 0.5% with rivaroxaban 20 mg, and 0.3% with aspirin.[29]

ADVERSE EFFECTS — The major adverse effect of all anticoagulants is bleeding, especially intracranial bleeding, which occurs about half as often with DOACs as it does with warfarin.[30] Nonbleeding adverse effects are summarized in Table 5.

DRUG INTERACTIONS — Many drugs can increase the risk of bleeding when coadministered with anticoagulants. Some drug interactions are listed in Table 5.

PRIMARY PREVENTION OF VTE — LMWH has been the most commonly recommended agent in guidelines for orthopedic and nonorthopedic surgery patients for whom postoperative prophylaxis is indicated.[31,32] Rivaroxaban and apixaban appear to be as effective as LMWH for prevention of VTE after knee or hip replacement surgery,[33,34] but the risk of bleeding may be higher with rivaroxaban.[35] In a double-blind trial, 3424 patients undergoing total hip or knee arthroplasty received once-daily rivaroxaban 10 mg for 5 days postoperatively and were then randomized to receive either rivaroxaban or aspirin 81 mg daily for an additional 9 days (total knee arthroplasty) or 30 days (total hip arthroplasty). Symptomatic VTE occurred in 0.64% of patients taking aspirin and in 0.70% of those taking rivaroxaban. Rates of major bleeding were 0.47% with aspirin and 0.29% with rivaroxaban. None of these differences were statistically significant.[36]

Table 5. Non-Bleeding Adverse Effects and Drug Interactions

Drug	Some Adverse Effects
Parenteral Anticoagulants	
Unfractionated heparin (UFH)	Heparin-induced thrombocytopenia, skin necrosis, urticaria, increased liver transaminases
Enoxaparin	Anemia, diarrhea, edema, confusion, nausea, thrombocytopenia, increased serum aminotransferases, injection-site reactions (pain, bleeding, hematoma), fever
Dalteparin	Thrombocytopenia, increased serum transaminases, injection-site reactions (pain, bleeding, hematoma), skin necrosis, fever, pruritus, rash
Desirudin	Deep vein thrombophlebitis, wound secretion, nausea, anemia, mass at injection sites
Fondaparinux	Anemia, hypotension, insomnia, dizziness, confusion, hypokalemia, purpura, thrombocytopenia, increased serum transaminases, epistaxis
Oral Anticoagulants	
Warfarin	Vasculitis, chills, alopecia, pruritus, urticaria, abdominal pain, bloating, nausea, vomiting, diarrhea, skin necrosis
Apixaban	Epistaxis, contusion, nausea, increased serum transaminases, anemia
Betrixaban	Epistaxis, UTI, constipation, hypokalemia, hypertension, headache, nausea, diarrhea
Dabigatran	Dyspepsia and gastritis-like symptoms
Edoxaban	Rash, abnormal liver function tests, anemia, epistaxis
Rivaroxaban	Abdominal pain, fatigue, back pain, muscle spasms, dizziness, anxiety, depression, insomnia, pruritus, wound secretion, UTI, increased serum transaminases

NSAIDs = nonsteroidal anti-inflammatory drugs; P-gp = P-glycoprotein; UTI = urinary tract infection
1. Drug interactions program from The Medical Letter. Available at: https://secure.medicalletter.org/druginteractions. Accessed March 1, 2018.
2. Acetaminophen, amiodarone, cefazolin, cefotetan, ceftriaxone, clarithromycin, fluconazole, fluoroquinolones, fluorouracil, fluoxetine, fluvastatin, fluvoxamine, metronidazole, phenytoin (initial use), rosuvastatin, trimethoprim-sulfamethoxazole, and voriconazole can increase the anticoagulant effect of warfarin. Barbiturates, carbamazepine, cholestyramine, colestipol, dicloxacillin, nafcillin, phenytoin, rifampin, St. John's wort, and sucralfate can decrease the anticoagulant effect of warfarin (Drug interactions from The Medical Letter. Available at: medicalletter.org/druginteractions. Accessed March 1, 2018.)

Some Drug Interactions[1]

Aspirin can increase the risk of bleeding/bruising; antiplatelet drugs can increase the risk of bleeding; NSAIDs can increase the anticoagulant effect; estrogens and progestins can reduce the anticoagulant effect; UFH, enoxaparin, and dalteparin may increase the hyperkalemic effects of ARBs, ACE inhibitors, potassium-sparing diuretics, aliskiren, and canagliflozin

Numerous drug and food interactions[2]

Substrate of CYP3A4 and P-gp; interacts with inhibitors and inducers of CYP3A4 and P-gp[3]; NSAIDs and other antiplatelet drugs can increase the risk of bleeding

Substrate of P-gp; interacts with inhibitors and inducers of P-gp[3]; NSAIDs and other antiplatelet drugs can increase the risk of bleeding

Substrate of P-gp; interacts with inhibitors and inducers of P-gp[3]; NSAIDs and other antiplatelet drugs can increase the risk of bleeding

Substrate of P-gp; interacts with inhibitors of P-gp[3]; should not be used with the P-gp inducer rifampin; NSAIDs and other antiplatelet drugs can increase the risk of bleeding

Substrate of CYP3A4 and P-gp; interacts with inhibitors and inducers of CYP3A4 and P-gp[3]; NSAIDs and other antiplatelet drugs can increase the risk of bleeding

3. Inhibitors and inducers of CYP enzymes and P-glycoprotein. Med Lett Drugs Ther 2017 September 18 (epub). Available at: medicalletter.org/downloads/CYP_PGP_Tables.pdf. Accessed March 1, 2018.

For prevention of VTE in patients hospitalized for an acute medical illness who are at increased risk of thrombosis, LMWH, low-dose UFH, or fondaparinux has been recommended.[37] Betrixaban, an oral, once-daily, direct factor Xa inhibitor, was recently approved by the FDA for this indication, based on the results of a clinical trial in which a composite endpoint of symptomatic DVT, asymptomatic proximal DVT detected by ultrasound, nonfatal PE, or VTE-related death occurred significantly less frequently at day 35 with 35-42 days of betrixaban than with 6-14 days of the LMWH enoxaparin.[38]

REVERSAL OF ANTICOAGULATION — In patients with serious bleeding caused by UFH or LMWH, IV infusion of protamine can reverse the anticoagulant effect. For patients with bleeding caused by warfarin, treatment with vitamin K can normalize the INR in 12-24 hours; for major bleeding, 4-factor prothrombin complex concentrate is recommended as well.[39] *Kcentra*, a human derived 4-factor prothrombin complex concentrate is approved by the FDA for urgent reversal of warfarin anticoagulation in adults with acute major bleeding.[40]

Until recently, there was no specific reversal agent for fondaparinux or for any of the DOACs. In 2015, the FDA approved idarucizumab *(Praxbind)*, a humanized monoclonal antibody fragment, for urgent reversal of the anticoagulant effect of the direct thrombin inhibitor dabigatran.[41] Idarucizumab rapidly decreases circulating levels of unbound dabigatran, neutralizing its anticoagulant effect within minutes. In a clinical trial, the median time to cessation of bleeding was ~2.5 hours.[42] Andexanet alfa *(Andexxa)*, a recombinant human factor Xa decoy protein that binds factor Xa inhibitors, is FDA-approved for urgent reversal of the anticoagulant effect of apixaban and rivaroxaban; in a clinical trial, a bolus and subsequent 2-hour infusion of the drug markedly reduced anti-factor Xa activity.[43,47]

The results of some studies indicate that the anticoagulant effects of DOACs can be reversed by prothrombin complex concentrates.[44,45] For life-threatening warfarin- or factor Xa-related bleeding, prothrombin complex concentrates are currently considered the best treatment option.

PREGNANCY — UFH has been used safely in pregnant women for many years. The large heparin molecule does not cross the placenta, and unlike warfarin, the drug is not teratogenic or toxic to the fetus. LMWH appears to be at least as safe and effective as UFH, and it is less likely to cause osteoporosis or heparin-induced thrombocytopenia[46]; the 2016 CHEST guidelines recommend use of LMWH during pregnancy. DOACs should not be used during pregnancy; some have caused fetal toxicity in animal studies. DOACs may be excreted in human breast milk and should be avoided in women who are breastfeeding.

1. C Kearon et al. Antithrombotic therapy for VTE disease: CHEST Guideline and Expert Panel Report. Chest 2016; 149:315.
2. A Jain and AS Cifu. Antithrombotic therapy for venous thromboembolic disease. JAMA 2017; 317:2008.
3. PS Wells et al. Treatment of venous thromboembolism. JAMA 2014; 311:717.
4. MB Streiff et al. Guidance for the treatment of deep vein thrombosis and pulmonary embolism. J Thromb Thrombolysis 2016; 41:32.
5. C Wall et al. Catheter-related thrombosis: a practical approach. J Intensive Care Soc 2016; 17:160.
6. SA Smith et al. How it all starts: initiation of the clotting cascade. Crit Rev Biochem Mol Biol 2015; 50:326.
7. New oral anticoagulants for acute venous thromboembolism. Med Lett Drugs Ther 2014; 56:3.
8. S Schulman et al. Dabigatran versus warfarin in the treatment of acute venous thromboembolism. N Engl J Med 2009; 361:2342.
9. S Schulman et al. Extended use of dabigatran, warfarin, or placebo in venous thromboembolism. N Engl J Med 2013; 368:709.
10. FDA Drug Safety Communication: FDA study of Medicare patients finds risks lower for stroke and death but higher for gastrointestinal bleeding with Pradaxa (dabigatran) compared to warfarin. Available at: www.fda.gov/Drugs/DrugSafety/ucm396470.htm. Accessed March 1, 2018.
11. Rivaroxaban (Xarelto) – a new oral anticoagulant. Med Lett Drugs Ther 2011; 53:65.
12. EINSTEIN Investigators et al. Oral rivaroxaban for symptomatic venous thromboembolism. N Engl J Med 2010; 363:2499.
13. EINSTEIN-PE Investigators et al. Oral rivaroxaban for the treatment of symptomatic pulmonary embolism. N Engl J Med 2012; 366:1287.
14. MR Lassen et al. Apixaban versus enoxaparin for thromboprophylaxis after knee replacement (ADVANCE-2): a randomised double-blind trial. Lancet 2010; 375:807.

15. MR Lassen et al. Apixaban versus enoxaparin for thromboprophylaxis after hip replacement. N Engl J Med 2010; 363:2487.
16. G Agnelli et al. Oral apixaban for the treatment of acute venous thromboembolism. N Engl J Med 2013; 369:799.
17. Hokusai-VTE Investigators et al. Edoxaban versus warfarin for the treatment of symptomatic venous thromboembolism. N Engl J Med 2013; 369:1406.
18. Betrixaban (Bevyxxa) for VTE prophylaxis in acute medical illness. Med Lett Drugs Ther 2018; 60:4.
19. N van Es et al. Direct oral anticoagulants compared with vitamin K antagonists for acute venous thromboembolism: evidence from phase 3 trials. Blood 2014; 124:1968.
20. N Kang and DM Sobieraj. Indirect treatment comparison of new oral anticoagulants for the treatment of acute venous thromboembolism. Thromb Res 2014; 133:1145.
21. AYY Lee et al. Tinzaparin vs warfarin for treatment of acute venous thromboembolism in patients with active cancer: a randomized clinical trial. JAMA 2015; 314:677.
22. GE Raskob et al. Edoxaban for the treatment of cancer-associated venous thromboembolism. N Engl J Med 2018; 378:615.
23. J Hirsh and JS Ginsberg. Edoxaban for the treatment of venous thromboembolism in patients with cancer. N Engl J Med 2018; 378:673.
24. K Uchino and AV Hernandez. Dabigatran association with higher risk of acute coronary events: meta-analysis of noninferiority randomized controlled trials. Arch Intern Med 2012; 172:397.
25. A Dhar et al. Anticoagulation in chronic liver disease. J Hepatol 2017; 66:1313.
26. C Becattini et al. Aspirin for preventing the recurrence of venous thromboembolism. N Engl J Med 2012; 366:1959.
27. TA Brighton et al. Low-dose aspirin for preventing recurrent venous thromboembolism. N Engl J Med 2012; 367:1979.
28. G Agnelli et al. Apixaban for extended treatment of venous thromboembolism. N Engl J Med 2013; 368:699.
29. JI Weitz et al. Rivaroxaban or aspirin for extended treatment of venous thromboembolism. N Engl J Med 2017; 376:1211.
30. Which oral anticoagulant for atrial fibrillation? Med Lett Drugs Ther 2016; 58:45.
31. Y Falck-Ytter et al. Prevention of VTE in orthopedic surgery patients: Antithrombotic Therapy and Prevention of Thrombosis, 9th ed: American College of Chest Physicians Evidence-Based Clinical Practice Guidelines. Chest 2012; 141:e325S.
32. MK Gould et al. Prevention of VTE in nonorthopedic surgical patients: Antithrombotic Therapy and Prevention of Thrombosis, 9th ed: American College of Chest Physicians Evidence-Based Clinical Practice Guidelines. Chest 2012; 141:e227S.
33. MR Lassen et al. Rivaroxaban versus enoxaparin for thromboprophylaxis after total knee arthroplasty. N Engl J Med 2008; 358:2776.
34. MR Lassen et al. Apixaban versus enoxaparin for thromboprophylaxis after hip replacement. N Engl J Med 2010; 363:2487.
35. BT Venker et al. Safety and efficacy of new anticoagulants for the prevention of venous thromboembolism after hip and knee arthroplasty: a meta-analysis. J Arthroplasty 2017; 32:645.

36. DR Anderson et al. Aspirin or rivaroxaban for VTE prophylaxis after hip or knee arthroplasty. N Engl J Med 2018; 378:699.
37. SR Kahn et al. Prevention of VTE in nonsurgical patients: Antithrombotic Therapy and Prevention of Thrombosis, 9th ed: American College of Chest Physicians Evidence-Based Clinical Practice Guidelines. Chest 2012; 141:e195S.
38. AT Cohen et al. Extended thromboprophylaxis with betrixaban in acutely ill medical patients. N Engl J Med 2016; 375:534.
39. S Christos and R Naples. Anticoagulation reversal and treatment strategies in major bleeding: update 2016. West J Emerg Med 2016; 17:264.
40. Kcentra: a 4-factor prothrombin complex concentrate for reversal of warfarin anticoagulation. Med Lett Drugs Ther 2013; 55:53.
41. Idarucizumab (Praxbind) - an antidote for dabigatran. Med Lett Drugs Ther 2015; 57:157.
42. CV Pollack Jr. et al. Idarucizumab for dabigatran reversal - full cohort analysis. N Engl J Med 2017; 377:431.
43. SJ Connolly et al. Andexanet alfa for acute major bleeding associated with factor Xa inhibitors. N Engl J Med 2016; 375:1131.
44. A Majeed et al. Management of rivaroxaban- or apixaban-associated major bleeding with prothrombin complex concentrates: a cohort study. Blood 2017; 130:1706.
45. JH Levy et al. Reversal agents for non-vitamin K antagonist oral anticoagulants. Nat Rev Cardiol 2018 Jan 18 (epub).
46. PS Gibson and R Powrie. Anticoagulants and pregnancy: when are they safe? Cleve Clin J Med 2009; 76:113.
47. Andexxa – an antidote for apixaban and rivaroxaban. Med Lett Drugs Ther 2018; 60:99.

DIET, DRUGS, DEVICES, AND SURGERY FOR
Weight Management

Original publication date – June 2018

Adults with a body mass index (BMI) between 25 and 29.9 kg/m^2 are considered overweight. Those with a BMI ≥30 are considered obese. The initial recommendation for any weight loss effort is to achieve a 5-10% reduction in weight, which has been associated with a reduction in the risk of developing type 2 diabetes, hypertension, and dyslipidemia. Diet, exercise, and behavior modification are the preferred methods for losing weight, but long-term weight maintenance can be difficult. Several drugs are FDA-approved for weight reduction and maintenance (see Table 1 on pages 258-261), and procedures such as endoscopic placement of dilated balloons have produced beneficial short-term results (see Table 2 on page 265), but bariatric surgery has been the most effective intervention for sustainable long-term weight loss and reduction of obesity-related comorbidities.[1]

LIFESTYLE INTERVENTIONS

DIET — Adults can lose 1-2 lbs (0.45-0.9 kg) per week by consuming 500-1000 fewer calories per day. A low-calorie diet typically reduces energy intake to 800-1500 calories daily. A very-low-calorie diet, which reduces intake to <800 calories daily, typically requires medical supervision, increases the risk of gallstones, and is recommended only for short-term weight loss. A meta-analysis of 6 randomized trials found that very-low-calorie diets did not produce greater long-term weight loss than conventional low-calorie diets.[2]

Recommendations for Weight Management
Lifestyle Interventions
▸ Diet, exercise, and behavior modification are the preferred methods for treatment of adults who are overweight or obese.
Drugs
▸ Pharmacologic therapy, which can produce short-term weight loss, should be reserved for patients with a BMI ≥30, or a BMI ≥27 and a weight-related co-morbidity such as hypertension, dyslipidemia, or type 2 diabetes. Phentermine/topiramate ER (*Qsymia*) is the most effective weight loss drug available to date.
Devices
▸ Devices such as the vagal blocking device, gastric aspiration device, and gastric balloons have produced short-term weight loss.
Surgery
▸ Bariatric surgery has been the most effective treatment for long-term weight loss and reduction of obesity-related comorbidities.

Weight-reduction diets that differ in macronutrient composition have been equally effective in achieving weight loss.[3] A randomized 2-year trial in 811 adults who were overweight compared 4 diets with the same degree of caloric restriction, but with varying proportions of protein (15 or 25%), fat (20 or 40%), and carbohydrate (35 to 65%). There were no significant differences between any of the groups in the amount of weight lost (about 4 kg).[4]

A meta-analysis of 48 randomized trials that included 7286 adults who were overweight or obese found no significant difference between a low-fat diet and a low-carbohydrate diet in the amount of weight lost at 6 and 12 months (about 8-9 kg at 6 months and 7-8 kg at 12 months).[5] In a randomized 12-month trial that compared a low-fat diet to a low-carbohydrate diet in 609 adults who were overweight or obese, there was no significant difference in weight lost between the two diets, and no association was observed between dietary effects on weight loss and hypothesized predisposing factors (genotype or baseline insulin secretion).[6]

Patients on a diet generally lose 5% of their initial weight over the first 6 months, but weight often returns to baseline over 2-3 years. The long-term ineffectiveness of weight-reduction diets may be due not only to poor adherence, but also to compensatory changes in energy expenditure that oppose maintenance of a lower body weight. It remains unclear whether macronutrient composition plays a role in weight maintenance; limited evidence suggests that high-protein, low-glycemic index diets may promote better long-term weight maintenance.[7]

BEHAVIORAL MODIFICATIONS — Guidelines for management of adults who are overweight or obese recommend at least monthly individual counseling sessions with a trained professional for one year to prevent weight regain.[8] In a randomized, controlled trial in 818 adults with a BMI ≥30, or a BMI ≥28 and an obesity-related comorbidity, 21% of those who followed a 6-month, 24-session, web-based nutritional advice/behavioral program with nursing support were successful in achieving and maintaining 5% weight loss at 12 months; addition of nurse support via phone or email increased the success rate to 32%.[9]

Extending the duration of behavioral interventions may result in more sustained weight loss; a formal, open-group, 52-week behavioral weight management program was significantly more effective than a 12-week program in maintaining weight loss at 1 year (loss of 6.8 kg vs 4.8 kg). The difference between the groups was still significant at 2 years.[10]

COMORBIDITIES — Lifestyle modification programs that focus on increased physical activity and changes in energy intake can reduce the risk of type 2 diabetes. In a trial in 3234 adults (mean age 51 years; mean BMI 34) with impaired glucose metabolism, lifestyle changes resulting in weight loss of 5.6 kg over approximately 3 years reduced the incidence of diabetes by 58%, compared to placebo.[11] Over a mean follow-up of 15 years after the initial trial, there was a 27% reduction in diabetes incidence in those who received lifestyle reinforcement semiannually, compared to placebo.[12]

In a randomized trial in 5145 adults with type 2 diabetes who were overweight or obese, intensive lifestyle intervention was more effective in achieving and maintaining significant weight loss (6.0% vs 3.5% with controls) and in improving A1C, blood pressure, HDL-cholesterol, and triglyceride levels, but not in reducing the incidence of cardiovascular events, compared to controls, at the end of the study (median follow-up of 9.6 years).[13]

DRUGS

Pharmacologic therapy should be reserved for adults with a BMI ≥30, or a BMI ≥27 and an obesity-related comorbidity such as hypertension, dyslipidemia, or type 2 diabetes. All weight-loss drugs are contraindicated for use during pregnancy. In patients with type 2 diabetes, use of weight loss-producing drugs can further reduce A1C by 0.3%-0.6%, compared to lifestyle modification alone.[14,15] However, weight loss increases insulin sensitivity and may increase the risk of hypoglycemia in patients with diabetes taking glucose-lowering medications (doses may need to be reduced).

SYMPATHOMIMETIC AMINES — The oldest weight-loss drugs are sympathomimetic amines such as phentermine (*Adipex-P*, and others) and diethylpropion, which are FDA-approved only for short-term use. Most studies of these drugs have reported an additional weight loss of only a fraction of a pound per week compared to placebo-treated patients.

Phentermine is available in combination with extended-release topiramate as *Qsymia*,[16] which is the most effective weight loss drug available to date; it has produced a dose-dependent mean weight loss of 6-13 kg over 56 weeks; 70% of patients treated with the higher dose of the drug (15/92 mg once/d) achieved ≥5% weight loss, with little weight regression back to baseline over 2 years of continuing to take the drug.[17-19] If ≥5% weight loss is not achieved after 12 weeks on the maximum dose, the drug should gradually be stopped; abrupt discontinuation of topiramate can cause seizures, even in patients with no history of epilepsy.

Adverse Effects – All sympathomimetic amines can increase heart rate and blood pressure and cause nervousness. Phentermine/topiramate can cause dry mouth, paresthesia, constipation, dysgeusia, and insomnia. Cognition, attention, concentration, and memory disturbances have been reported. Phentermine is contraindicated for use in patients with cardiovascular disease, hyperthyroidism, glaucoma, or a history of drug abuse. It should not be used with or within 14 days of a monoamine oxidase inhibitor (MAOI). Topiramate is a carbonic anhydrase inhibitor and can cause metabolic acidosis, which increases the risk of renal stones. *Qsymia* is a schedule IV controlled substance and is only available through a voluntary REMS program designed to prevent use in pregnancy.

ORLISTAT — Available both over the counter *(Alli)* and by prescription *(Xenical)*, orlistat is a pancreatic and gastric lipase inhibitor that decreases GI absorption of fat. When used as an adjunct to diet, it is modestly effective in increasing weight loss. Patients taking orlistat 120 mg three times daily for 1-4 years have lost about 3 kg more than those taking placebo.[20]

Adverse Effects – Flatulence with discharge, oily spotting, and fecal urgency occur predominantly after consumption of high-fat foods and are associated with a high incidence of drug discontinuation. Severe liver injury has been reported rarely, but no cause-and-effect relationship has been established. Orlistat increases oxalate absorption and may increase the risk of developing calcium oxalate renal stones. Because the drug reduces absorption of fat-soluble vitamins, patients taking orlistat should also take a multivitamin daily at bedtime.[21] Levothyroxine should be taken 4 hours before or after taking orlistat.

LORCASERIN — A schedule IV controlled substance, lorcaserin *(Belviq, Belviq XR)* is a selective serotonin $5\text{-}HT_{2C}$ receptor agonist that suppresses appetite. It is only modestly effective for weight loss, but is generally well tolerated. In clinical trials, <50% of adults taking the drug lost ≥5% of their baseline weight; the average placebo-corrected weight loss after one year of use has been about 3%.[1] Patients who do not lose ≥5% of their baseline weight by 12 weeks should stop taking lorcaserin.

Table 1. Some FDA-Approved Drugs for Weight Management[1]	
Drug	**Some Available Formulations**
Sympathomimetic Amines	
Benzphetamine − generic	50 mg tabs
Diethylpropion − generic	25 mg tabs
extended-release − generic	75 mg ER tabs
Phendimetrazine − generic	35 mg tabs;
extended-release − generic	105 mg ER caps
Phentermine[5] − generic	15, 30, 37.5 mg caps; 37.5 mg tabs
Adipex-P (Teva)	37.5 mg tabs, caps
Lomaira (KVK-Tech)	8 mg tabs
Sympathomimetic Amine/Antiepileptic Combination	
Phentermine/topiramate ER −	7.5/46, 15/92 mg ER caps[6]
Qsymia (Vivus)	
Lipase Inhibitor	
Orlistat − Xenical (Chepla)	120 mg caps
Alli[11] (GSK)	60 mg caps
Serotonin Receptor Agonist	
Lorcaserin − Belviq (Eisai)	10 mg tabs
extended-release −	
Belviq XR	20 mg ER tabs

ER = extended-release
1. Weight loss drugs, including over-the-counter medications, are not recommended for use during pregnancy.
2. Placebo-corrected weight loss above diet and lifestyle modifications alone.
3. Approximate WAC for 30 days' treatment at the lowest usual adult dosage. WAC = wholesaler acquisition cost or manufacturer's published price to wholesalers; WAC represents a published catalogue or list price and may not represent an actual transactional price. Source: AnalySource® Monthly. May 5, 2018. Reprinted with permission by First Databank, Inc. All rights reserved. ©2018. www.fdbhealth.com/policies/drug-pricing-policy.
4. Only approved for short-term use (a few weeks). Most studies have reported an additional weight loss of only a fraction of a pound per week compared to placebo-treated patients.
5. Phentermine was widely used with fenfluramine until the combination ("phen-fen") was found to be associated with heart valve abnormalities. Fenfluramine has been withdrawn from the market.
6. Also available in 3.75/23 mg and 11.25/69 mg capsules which are intended for use only during titration.
7. If ≥5% weight loss is not achieved after 12 weeks on the maximum dose, the drug should be discontinued. Phentermine/topiramate ER and bupropion/naltrexone should be gradually discontinued.

Usual Adult Dosage	Mean Weight Loss[2]/ % Patients with Weight Loss ≥5%	Cost[3]
25-50 mg once/d-tid	See Footnote 4	$37.50
25 mg tid	See Footnote 4	20.10
75 mg once/d		25.30
35 mg bid or tid	See Footnote 4	8.20
105 mg once/d		32.30
15-37.5 mg once/d	See Footnote 4	16.00
37.5 mg once/d	See Footnote 4	62.40
8 mg tid	See Footnote 4	43.50
7.5/46-15/92 mg once/d[7]	4.1-10.7 kg/45-70%[8-10]	
		186.00
120 mg tid	2.5-3.4 kg/35-73%[12]	586.10
60 mg tid		44.00
10 mg bid[7]	2.9-3.6 kg/38-48%[13-15]	264.90
20 mg once/d[7]		264.90

8. DB Allison et al. Controlled-release phentermine/topiramate in severely obese adults: a randomized controlled trial (EQUIP). Obesity 2012; 20:330.
9. KM Gadde et al. Effects of low-dose, controlled-release, phentermine plus topiramate combination on weight and associated comorbidities in overweight and obese adults (CONQUER): a randomised, placebo-controlled, phase 3 trial. Lancet 2011; 377:1341.
10. The range includes weight loss observed with titration and maintenance dosages.
11. Available over the counter.
12. SZ Yanovski and JA Yanovski. Long-term drug treatment for obesity: a systematic and clinical review. JAMA 2014; 311:74.
13. SR Smith et al. Multicenter, placebo-controlled trial of lorcaserin for weight management. N Engl J Med 2010; 363:245.
14. MC Fidler et al. A one-year randomized trial of lorcaserin for weight loss in obese and overweight adults: the BLOSSOM trial. J Clin Endocrinol Metab 2011; 96:3067.
15. PM O'Neil et al. Randomized placebo-controlled clinical trial of lorcaserin for weight loss in type 2 diabetes mellitus: the BLOOM-DM study. Obesity 2012; 20:1426.

Continued on next page

Table 1. Some FDA-Approved Drugs for Weight Management[1] (continued)	
Drug	**Some Available Formulations**
Opioid Antagonist/Antidepressant Combination	
Naltrexone/bupropion – *Contrave* (Orexigen)	8/90 mg ER tabs
Glucagon-Like Peptide-1 (GLP-1) Receptor Agonist	
Liraglutide – *Saxenda* (Novo Nordisk)	18 mg/3 mL prefilled pen[19]

ER = extended-release
16. FL Greenway et al. Effect of naltrexone plus bupropion on weight loss in overweight and obese adults (COR-I): a multicentre, randomised, double-blind, placebo-controlled, phase 3 trial. Lancet 2010; 376:595.
17. CM Apovian et al. A randomized, phase 3 trial of naltrexone SR/bupropion SR on weight and obesity-related risk factors (COR-II). Obesity 2013; 21:935.
18. A Wadden et al. Weight loss with naltrexone SR/bupropion SR combination therapy as an adjunct to behavior modification: the COR-BMOD trial. Obesity 2011; 19:110.

Adverse Effects – Lorcaserin can cause headache, nausea, dizziness, euphoria, and impairment of attention and cognition. The labeling includes a warning about the possibility of cardiac valvulopathy (it did not occur significantly more frequently with lorcaserin than with placebo in clinical trials) because agonism of the 5-HT_{2C} receptor was implicated in cardiac valvulopathy associated with fenfluramine. Serotonin syndrome has been reported; lorcaserin is not recommended for use with other serotonergic drugs, such as selective serotonin reuptake inhibitors (SSRIs) or serotonin-norepinephrine reuptake inhibitors (SNRIs), or with drugs that impair serotonin metabolism, such as MAOIs.

BUPROPION/NALTREXONE — The dopamine/norepinepherine reuptake inhibitor bupropion (*Wellbutrin SR, Zyban*, and others) and the opioid receptor antagonist naltrexone are available in a fixed-dose combination *(Contrave)* that is FDA-approved for weight management. In 4 clinical trials, bupropion/naltrexone was associated with ≥5% weight loss in 39-66% of patients after 56 weeks. Placebo-corrected weight loss at the end of 56 weeks was 3-5% in the largest trials.[22] If ≥5% weight

Usual Adult Dosage	Mean Weight Loss[2]/ % Patients with Weight Loss ≥5%	Cost[3]
16/180 mg bid[7]	3.7-5.2 kg/39-66%[10,16-18]	$278.00
3 mg SC once/d	3.7-5.8 kg/44-62%[10,20,21]	1200.40

19. Each pen can deliver doses of 0.6, 1.2, 1.8, 2.4, or 3 mg. Sold in packages containing 3 or 5 multi-dose pens.
20. A Astrup et al. Safety, tolerability and sustained weight loss over 2 years with the once-daily human GLP-1 analog, liraglutide. Int J Obes (Lond) 2012; 36:843.
21. TA Wadden et al. Weight maintenance and additional weight loss with liraglutide after low-calorie-diet-induced weight loss: The SCALE Maintenance randomized study. Int J Obes (Lond) 2015; 39:187.

loss is not achieved after 12 weeks at the maintenance dosage, the drug should gradually be stopped.

Adverse Effects – Bupropion/naltrexone can cause nausea, vomiting, headache, constipation, dizziness, and dry mouth. The labeling includes a boxed warning about suicidal thoughts and behavior associated with use of antidepressants and serious neuropsychiatric reactions reported with use of bupropion for smoking cessation; clinical trials of bupropion/naltrexone did not find an association with suicidality. Bupropion may lower the seizure threshold and can cause CNS depression; additive effects could occur when bupropion is used concomitantly with other drugs that increase seizure risk or cause CNS depression. Increases in heart rate and blood pressure have been reported in patients taking bupropion; the drug is not recommended for use in patients with uncontrolled blood pressure. Aminotransferase elevations and hepatotoxicity have been reported in patients taking naltrexone.

LIRAGLUTIDE — The once-daily injectable glucagon-like peptide-1 (GLP-1) receptor agonist liraglutide, which is FDA-approved for treatment of type 2 diabetes as *Victoza*,[23] is also approved for weight loss as *Saxenda*. GLP-1 receptor agonists delay gastric emptying and cause satiety.[24]

In a 56-week, randomized, double-blind trial in 3731 patients with a mean BMI of 38.3, use of liraglutide 3 mg daily resulted in a placebo-corrected weight loss of 5.6 kg; 63% of patients taking the drug lost ≥5% of their baseline weight.[25]

In a 3-year, randomized, double-blind trial in 1128 patients with prediabetes, use of liraglutide 3 mg/day resulted in a placebo-corrected weight loss of 4.3% and a significant reduction in development of type 2 diabetes (2% of patients on liraglutide vs 6% on placebo).[26]

Adverse Effects – Liraglutide can cause nausea, diarrhea, constipation, vomiting, hypoglycemia, decreased appetite, and dyspepsia. Acute pancreatitis, cholelithiasis, acute renal failure, and increased heart rate have also been reported. Serious hypersensitivity reactions including angioedema and anaphylaxis have occurred. Thyroid C-cell tumors have been reported in rodents given liraglutide; the labeling includes a boxed warning about the risk of these tumors. The drug is contraindicated in patients with a personal or family history of medullary thyroid carcinoma and in those with Multiple Endocrine Neoplasia syndrome type 2 (MEN 2).

DEVICES

VAGAL BLOCKING DEVICE — The *Maestro Rechargeable System* is a subcutaneously implanted, rechargeable, neuroregulator device that blocks vagus nerve signals between the stomach and the brain to enhance satiety and decrease food intake.[27] It is FDA-approved for use in adults with a BMI of 40-45, or a BMI ≥35 and at least one obesity-related comorbidity who have been unable to lose weight with a weight loss program for 5 years. The device is implanted laparoscopically in the thoracic side wall. It contains two electrodes, placed onto the anterior and posterior vagal nerve trunks above the gastroesophageal junction, that are programmed to deliver intermittent high-frequency electrical pulses, which block vagus nerve signals, for 9-13 daytime hours.

Two clinical trials have compared the *Maestro* device to a sham device. In one trial in 294 patients, there was no significant difference in weight lost between the treatment and sham group, possibly because some patients used the *Maestro* device ≤9 hours per day.[28] In a second trial in 239 patients, mean excess weight loss was 24.4% ("excess weight" is the weight above the weight at a BMI of 25) with active treatment, compared to 15.9% with sham treatment, an 8.5% difference that did not reach the prespecified superiority margin of 10%.[29]

Adverse Effects – Pain at the neuroregulator site occurred in about 40% of actively-treated patients. Heartburn/dyspepsia, nausea, dysphagia, eructation, and abdominal pain also occurred. Serious adverse events that required longer hospitalizations occurred in 9% of actively-treated patients and in none of the sham controls.[29]

GASTRIC ASPIRATION DEVICE — The *AspireAssist* device permits patients to drain a portion of their stomach contents into a toilet after each meal, reducing the amount of absorbed calories by about 30%. It is FDA-approved for adults ≥22 years old with a BMI of 35-55 who are unable to achieve and maintain weight loss through nonsurgical programs.[30] The device consists of a tube inserted endoscopically, similar to a percutaneous endoscopic gastrostomy (PEG) feeding tube, a port valve, a drainage tube with a clamp, and water reservoir that allows patients to flush the tube and stomach with potable water. The process takes 5-10 minutes to complete. In a 52-week, open-label trial comparing *Aspire-Assist* plus lifestyle counseling with lifestyle counseling alone, use of the device was associated with a 31.5% loss of excess weight compared to a 9.8% loss in the control group.

Adverse Effects – Abdominal pain, nausea and vomiting, electrolyte disturbances, and peristomal granulation tissue and irritation at the tube site are common.[31]

GASTRIC BALLOON DEVICES — Three gastric balloon devices *(Obalon Balloon System; Orbera Intragastric Balloon System*; *ReShape Integrated Dual Balloon System)* are FDA-approved for up to 6 months' use in adults with a BMI of 30-40 who have been unable to lose or maintain weight with diet and exercise (use of *ReShape* also requires the presence of one obesity-related comorbidity). The *ReShape* and *Orbera* devices are endoscopically-inserted gastric balloons; *Orbera* is a single balloon filled with saline and *ReShape* is a double balloon filled with saline and methylene blue. The *Obalon Balloon System* uses up to three deflated balloons swallowed at ≥14 day intervals (during the first 3 months) as capsules attached to an inflation catheter. The catheter is used to inflate the balloons, without endoscopy or sedation, with nitrogen/sulfur hexafluoride gas and is then withdrawn.

All of these devices are left in place for 6 months and then deflated and removed endoscopically. In general, they increase satiety/fullness and produce a mean excess weight loss of about 25-30%.[32,33] They have not been compared directly to one another or to pharmacologic or surgical methods of weight loss.

Adverse Effects – The balloon devices are contraindicated for use in patients with a wide variety of GI conditions, including prior GI or weight reduction surgery, inflammatory bowel disease, obstructive disorders, GI ulcers, intestinal varices, stricture or stenosis, severe reflux, prior GI bleeding, and coagulopathy. All three devices are associated with nausea, emesis, abdominal pain, reflux symptoms, and abdominal distention/bloating. If they deflate and migrate, they can cause GI obstruction. Gastric ulceration and esophageal perforation can occur. The long-term safety of gastric balloon devices for weight loss is unknown; deaths have occurred.[34]

BARIATRIC SURGERY

Surgical treatment for obesity is generally limited to patients with a BMI ≥40, or a BMI ≥35 with an obesity-related comorbidity. A study from the

Table 2. Gastric Balloons for Weight Loss		
Device	Mean Excess Weight Lost[1]	Mean Weight Regained[2]
Obalon Balloon System[3] (Obalon)	24.1% (14.4 lbs)	~12.5% (1.8 lbs)
Orbera Intragastric Balloon System[4] (Apollo Endosurgery)	26.5% (19.4 lbs)	~28.9% (5.6 lbs)
ReShape Integrated Dual Balloon System[4] (ReShape Medical)	27.9% (15.9 lbs)	~34.0% (5.4 lbs)

1. Defined as weight above the weight at a BMI of 25 kg/m^2. For *Orbera*, results at 36 weeks; for *ReShape* and *Obalon*, results at 24 weeks.
2. 6 months after removal of the balloons.
3. Obalon Balloon System - another gastric balloon for weight loss. Med Lett Drugs Ther 2017; 59:102.
4. ReShape and Orbera - two gastric balloon devices for weight loss. Med Lett Drugs Ther 2015; 57:122.

American College of Surgeons National Surgical Quality Improvement Program database noted a large shift away from procedures that cause malabsorption such as Roux-en-Y gastric bypass (58% of procedures in 2010; 38% in 2014), and towards restrictive procedures such as sleeve gastrectomy (9% of procedures in 2010; 58% in 2014).[35]

LAPAROSCOPIC ADJUSTABLE GASTRIC BANDING — An adjustable gastric band placed laparoscopically around the proximal portion of the stomach and injected with variable amounts of saline to promote restriction is generally felt to be the safest, but least effective, of the current bariatric surgery procedures. Its use has declined from 29% of bariatric surgery procedures in 2010 to 3% in 2014.[35]

Efficacy – A prospective cohort study of laparoscopic adjustable gastric banding in 3227 patients found a mean excess weight loss of 47% at ≥10 years.[36]

Adverse Effects – Laparoscopic adjustable gastric banding is a restrictive procedure with no associated malabsorption. In the prospective cohort study in >3000 patients followed for ≥10 years, there was no perioperative mortality associated with placement of a laparoscopic adjustable gastric band. Slippage, band erosion, excess vomiting, and port-site and tubing problems are the most common adverse effects; these may require an operative revision.

SLEEVE GASTRECTOMY — Sleeve gastrectomy is a laparoscopic partial gastrectomy in which most of the greater curvature of the stomach is removed, resulting in a tubular stomach. Although originally considered a bridge to another type of bariatric procedure, sleeve gastrectomy is now done as a primary procedure.

Efficacy – A review of 20 studies of sleeve gastrectomy with results reported at least 5 years post-procedure found a mean excess weight loss of 58% at 5 years; the percentage of patients with resolution or improvement of a comorbid condition was 78% for type 2 diabetes, 68% for hypertension, and 66% for dyslipidemia.[37]

Adverse Effects – Sleeve gastrectomy is a restrictive procedure that also may affect intestinal hormone regulation. In some studies, it had a shorter mean operative time than gastric bypass, a lower 30-day reoperation rate, and a lower risk-adjusted 30-day serious morbidity rate, with equivalent 30-day mortality.[38]

ROUX-EN-Y GASTRIC BYPASS (RYGB) — A mixed restrictive and malabsorptive procedure, RYGB creates a proximal 20-30 mL pouch of stomach and anastomoses it to a limb of jejunum, bypassing most of the stomach, all of the duodenum, and the first 15-20 cm of the jejunum. Undigested nutrients meet digestive enzymes in the common channel where the two separated limbs join.

Efficacy – In a single institution report on 651 RYGB patients (335 open procedures and 316 laparoscopies) with a 10-year follow-up, the reduction in excess weight peaked at 74% by year 2 and was 52% at year 10. Obesity-related complications were also significantly reduced at year 10.[39] In a trial in 1156 patients with severe obesity, mean weight loss was 45.0 kg at 2 years and 35.0 kg at 12 years in patients who had an RYGB, compared to 0-3 kg at 12 years in those who did not have surgery. Patients who had an RYGB also had lower rates of type 2 diabetes, hypertension, and dyslipidemia at 12 years.[40]

Adverse Effects – Iron, calcium, folate, vitamin D, and vitamin B_{12} deficiencies can occur with RYGB because of malabsorption. Rapid emptying from the gastric pouch into the jejunum can cause dumping syndrome (nausea, bloating, colic, diarrhea). Some patients who had an RYGB developed clinically significant hyperinsulinemic hypoglycemia; the mechanism remains unclear.[41]

BILIOPANCREATIC DIVERSION — Biliopancreatic diversion with duodenal switch (BPD/DS) combines a restrictive procedure similar to sleeve gastrectomy with a procedure that bypasses about three quarters of the small intestine. It results in greater weight loss ($\geq$70% excess weight loss) than other procedures, but has higher risks of complications and death.

COMPARATIVE STUDIES — In an open-label trial (SLEEVEPASS) in 240 extremely obese patients (mean BMI of 45.9) randomized to laparoscopic sleeve gastrectomy or RYGB, mean excess weight loss at 5 years was less with sleeve gastrectomy than with RYGB (49% vs 57%).[42]

In a randomized trial (SM-BOSS) in 217 patients with extreme obesity (mean BMI of 43.9), there was no significant difference in excess weight loss at 5 years with sleeve gastrectomy (61.1%) compared to RYGB (68.3%). The reoperation rate with sleeve gastrectomy, mostly for GERD symptoms, was lower than with RYGB (16% vs 22%); reoperation for RYGB was most often for internal hernia repair. At year 5, the complete or partial remission rate for type 2 diabetes was 67.9% with RYGB and 66.5% with sleeve gastrectomy, and the percentage of patients who stopped medication for dyslipidemia was 60% with RYGB and 47% with sleeve gastrectomy. None of these differences were statistically significant, but significantly more patients who had an RYGB were able to stop antihypertensive medications at 5 years (51% vs 29% with sleeve gastrectomy). Five-year morbidity rates were 19% for sleeve gastrectomy and 26% for RYGB. There was no significant difference in quality of life.[43]

In a 7-year follow-up study of 2348 patients (mean BMI of 47) who had bariatric surgery, rates of weight loss were higher with RYGB than with LAGB (28.4% vs 15%); rates of weight regain were low in both groups (3.9% and 1.4%, respectively). Both groups achieved a reduction in dyslipidemia, but only the RYGB patients had a sustained reduction in the incidence of type 2 diabetes and hypertension.[44]

IN DIABETES — In a prospective trial in 60 patients with type 2 diabetes and a mean BMI of 45, 75% of patients who had an RYGB had complete remission of their diabetes, compared to none of those who received conventional medical therapy.[45]

In a 1-year trial in 150 patients with type 2 diabetes and a mean BMI of 36, RYGB and sleeve gastrectomy were associated with weight loss of 29 kg and 25 kg and diabetes remission rates of 42% and 37%, respectively, compared to weight loss of 5.4 kg and a diabetes remission rate of 12% with intensive medical therapy.[46] In a 5-year follow-up of this cohort (baseline BMI of 37 for those that completed 5 years), weight loss was 23% with RYGB and 19% with sleeve gastrectomy, and 29% of patients who had an RYGB and 23% of those who had a sleeve gastrectomy achieved an A1C of $\leq 6\%$, compared to only 5% of those who received intensive medical therapy.[47]

In a 5-year observational follow-up of a 2-year randomized trial in 120 patients with type 2 diabetes, all of whom had received intensive lifestyle and medical management and 50% had undergone RYGB, a composite outcome of A1C <7%, LDL <100 mg/dL, and systolic blood pressure <130 mm Hg was achieved in 23% of RYGB patients, compared to 4% of those who received only lifestyle and medical management. At 5 years, diabetes remission had occurred in 16% of RYGB patients compared to 5% of those in the control group.[48]

MORTALITY — In a 10-year observational cohort study in 4047 obese patients, mortality (adjusted for sex, age, and risk factors) was 29% lower in patients who had bariatric surgery than in matched controls who received conventional treatment. Bariatric surgery was also associated with fewer cardiovascular deaths (HR 0.47) and first-time cardiovascular events (HR 0.67).[49] In a retrospective cohort study comparing 8385 patients (median BMI of 40.6) who had bariatric surgery (3635 laparoscopic banding, 1388 RYGB, and 3362 laparoscopic sleeve gastrectomy) with 25,155 BMI-matched patients who received standard treatment over a period of about 4.5 years, all-cause mortality was significantly lower in the surgical group (1.3% vs 2.3%).[50]

1. CM Apovian et al. Pharmacological management of obesity: an Endocrine Society clinical practice guideline. J Clin Endocrinol Metab 2015; 100:342.
2. AG Tsai and TA Wadden. The evolution of very-low-calorie diets: an update and meta-analysis. Obesity 2006; 14:1283.
3. MD Jensen et al. 2013 AHA/ACC/TOS guideline for the management of overweight and obesity in adults: a report of the American College of Cardiology/American Heart Association Task Force on Practice Guidelines and The Obesity Society. Circulation 2014; 129:S102.
4. FM Sacks et al. Comparison of weight-loss diets with different compositions of fat, protein, and carbohydrates. N Engl J Med 2009; 360:859.
5. BC Johnston et al. Comparison of weight loss among named diet programs in overweight and obese adults: a meta-analysis. JAMA 2014; 312:923.
6. CD Gardner et al. Effect of low-fat vs low-carbohydrate diet on 12-month weight loss in overweight adults and the association with genotype pattern or insulin secretion: the DIETFITS randomized clinical trial. JAMA 2018; 319:667.
7. TM Larsen et al. Diets with high or low protein content and glycemic index for weight-loss maintenance. N Engl J Med 2010; 363:2102.
8. VL Webb and TA Wadden. Intensive lifestyle intervention for obesity: principles, practices, and results. Gastroenterology 2017; 152:1752.
9. P Little et al. An internet-based intervention with brief nurse support to manage obesity in primary care (POWeR+): a pragmatic, parallel-group, randomised controlled trial. Lancet Diabetes Endocrinol 2016; 4:821.
10. AL Ahern et al. Extended and standard duration weight-loss programme referrals for adults in primary care (WRAP): a randomised controlled trial. Lancet 2017; 389:2214.
11. WC Knowler et al. Reduction in the incidence of type 2 diabetes with lifestyle intervention or metformin. N Engl J Med 2002; 346:393.
12. Diabetes Prevention Program Research Group. Long-term effects of lifestyle intervention or metformin on diabetes development and microvascular complications over 15-year follow-up: the Diabetes Prevention Program Outcomes Study. Lancet Diabetes Endocrinol 2015; 3:866.
13. Look AHEAD Research Group et al. Cardiovascular effects of intensive lifestyle intervention in type 2 diabetes. N Engl J Med 2013; 369:145.

14. P Hollander et al. Effects of naltrexone sustained-release/bupropion sustained-release combination therapy on body weight and glycemic parameters in overweight and obese patients with type 2 diabetes. Diabetes Care 2013; 36:4022.

15. WT Garvey et al. Weight-loss therapy in type 2 diabetes: effects of phentermine and topiramate extended release. Diabetes Care 2014; 37:3309.

16. Two drugs for weight loss. Med Lett Drugs Ther 2012; 54:69.

17. DB Allison et al. Controlled-release phentermine/topiramate in severely obese adults: a randomized controlled trial (EQUIP). Obesity 2012; 20:330.

18. KM Gadde et al. Effects of low-dose, controlled-release, phentermine plus topiramate combination on weight and associated comorbidities in overweight and obese adults (CONQUER): a randomised, placebo-controlled, phase 3 trial. Lancet 2011; 377:1341.

19. WT Garvey et al. Two-year sustained weight loss and metabolic benefits with controlled-release phentermine/topiramate in obese and overweight adults (SEQUEL): a randomized, placebo-controlled, phase 3 extension study. Am J Clin Nutr 2012; 95:297.

20. SZ Yanovski and JA Yanovski. Long-term drug treatment for obesity: a systematic and clinical review. JAMA 2014; 311:74.

21. KM Gadde et al. Obesity: pathophysiology and management. J Am Coll Cardiol 2018; 71: 69.

22. Contrave – a combination of bupropion and naltrexone for weight loss. Med Lett Drugs Ther 2014; 56:112.

23. Liraglutide (Victoza) for type 2 diabetes. Med Lett Drugs Ther 2010; 52:25.

24. Liraglutide (Saxenda) for weight loss. Med Lett Drugs Ther 2015; 57:89.

25. X Pi-Sunyer et al. A randomized, controlled trial of 3.0 mg of liraglutide in weight management. N Engl J Med 2015; 373:11.

26. CW le Roux et al. 3 years of liraglutide versus placebo for type 2 diabetes risk reduction and weight management in individuals with prediabetes: a randomised, double-blind trial. Lancet 2017; 389:1399.

27. Maestro rechargeable system for weight loss. Med Lett Drugs Ther 2016; 58:54.

28. MG Sarr et al. The EMPOWER study: randomized, prospective, double-blind, multicenter trial of vagal blockade to induce weight loss in morbid obesity. Obes Surg 2012; 22:1771.

29. S Ikramuddin et al. Effect of reversible intermittent intra-abdominal vagal nerve blockade on morbid obesity: the ReCharge randomized clinical trial. JAMA 2014; 312:915.

30. AspireAssist - A new device for weight loss. Med Lett Drugs Ther 2016; 58:109.

31. CC Thompson et al. Percutaneous gastrostomy device for the treatment of class II and class III obesity: results of a randomized controlled trial. Am J Gastroenterol 2017; 112:447.

32. Obalon Balloon System - another gastric balloon for weight loss. Med Lett Drugs Ther 2017; 59:102.

33. ReShape and Orbera - two gastric balloon devices for weight loss. Med Lett Drugs Ther 2015; 57:122.

34. FDA Update: Potential risks with liquid-filled intragastric balloons – letter to health care providers. Available at: www.fda.gov/MedicalDevices/Safety/LetterstoHealthCareProviders/ucm570707.htm. Accessed May 24, 2018.

35. Z Khorgami et al. Trends in utilization of bariatric surgery, 2010-2014: sleeve gastrectomy dominates. Surg Obes Relat Dis 2017; 13:774.

36. PE O'Brien et al. Long-term outcomes after bariatric surgery: fifteen-year follow-up of adjustable gastric banding and a systematic review of the bariatric surgical literature. Ann Surg 2013; 257:87.

37. Z Juodeikis and G Brimas. Long-term results after sleeve gastrectomy: a systematic review. Surg Obes Relat Dis 2017; 13:693.

38. MT Young et al. Use and outcomes of laparoscopic sleeve gastrectomy vs laparoscopic gastric bypass: analysis of the American College of Surgeons NSQIP. J Am Coll Surg 2015; 220:880.

39. JH Mehaffey et al. 10-year outcomes after roux-en-Y gastric bypass. Ann Surg 2016; 264:121.

40. TD Adams et al. Weight and metabolic outcomes 12 years after gastric bypass. N Engl J Med 2017; 377:1143.

41. GJ Service et al. Hyperinsulinemic hypoglycemia with nesidioblastosis after gastric-bypass surgery. N Engl J Med 2005; 353:249.

42. P Salminen et al. Effect of laparoscopic sleeve gastrectomy vs laparoscopic roux-en-y gastric bypass on weight loss at 5 years among patients with morbid obesity: the SLEEVEPASS randomized clinical trial. JAMA 2018; 319:241.

43. R Peterli et al. Effect of laparoscopic sleeve gastrectomy vs laparoscopic roux-en-y gastric bypass on weight loss in patients with morbid obesity: the SM-BOSS randomized clinical trial. JAMA 2018; 319:255.

44. AP Courcoulas et al. Seven-year weight trajectories and health outcomes in the longitudinal assessment of bariatric surgery (LABS) study. JAMA Surg 2017 Dec 6 (epub).

45. G Mingrone et al. Bariatric surgery versus conventional medical therapy for type 2 diabetes. N Engl J Med 2012; 366:1577.

46. PR Schauer et al. Bariatric surgery versus intensive medical therapy in obese patients with diabetes. N Engl J Med 2012; 366:1567.

47. PR Schauer et al. Bariatric surgery versus intensive medical therapy for diabetes – 5-year outcomes. N Engl J Med 2017; 376:641.

48. S Ikramuddin et al. Lifestyle intervention and medical management with vs without roux-en-y gastric bypass and control of hemoglobin A1c, LDL cholesterol, and systolic blood pressure at 5 years in the diabetes surgery study. JAMA 2018; 319:266.

49. L Sjöström et al. Bariatric surgery and long-term cardiovascular events. JAMA 2012; 307:56.

50. O Reges et al. Association of bariatric surgery using laparoscopic banding, roux-en-y gastric bypass, or laparoscopic sleeve gastrectomy vs usual care obesity management with all-cause mortality. JAMA 2018; 319:279.

Index

Index

Index

Index

Index

Index

Index